JUNK
FOOD
TO
REAL
FOOD

KEATS TITLES OF RELATED INTEREST

Kitchen Magic ■ LINDA WEISS

Round-the-World Cooking at the Natural Gourmet ■ DEBRA STARK

Grain Power ■ BEATRICE TRUM HUNTER

Nutrition and Physical Degeneration ■ WESTON A. PRICE, D.D.S.

The Family Wholegrain Baking Book ■ BEATRICE TRUM HUNTER

Add a Few Sprouts ■ MARTHA H. OLIVER

The Book of Raw Fruit and Vegetable Juices and Drinks ■ WILLIAM H. LEE, R.PH., PH.D.

Cooking with Mrs. Appleyard ■ LOUISE ANDREWS KENT
ELIZABETH KENT GAY

The Wholegrain Health-Saver Cookbook ■ MIRIAM POLUNIN

Diet and Disease ■ E. CHERASKIN, M.D., D.M.D.
W.M. RINGSDORF, JR., D.M.D.
J.W. CLARK, D.D.S.

Eating for Health and Happiness ■ ESTHER L. SMITH

Healthier Children ■ BARBARA KAHAN

JUNK FOOD TO REAL FOOD

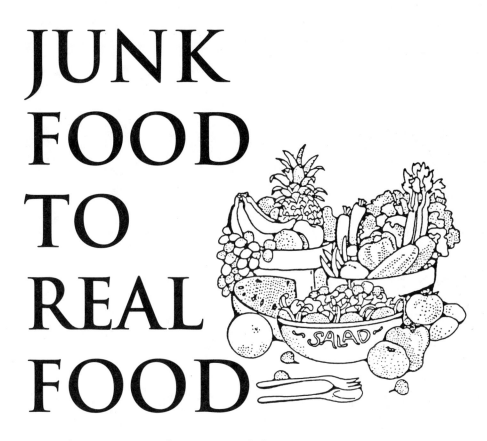

A Blueprint for Healthier Eating

CAROL A. NOSTRAND

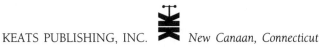

KEATS PUBLISHING, INC. *New Canaan, Connecticut*

Junk Food to Real Food is not intended as medical advice. Its intent is solely informational and educational. Please consult a health professional should a need for one be indicated.

JUNK FOOD TO REAL FOOD: A Blueprint for Healthier Eating

Library of Congress Cataloging-in-Publication Data

Nostrand, Carol A.
   Junk food to real food : a blueprint for healthier eating / Carol
A. Nostrand.
     p.   cm.
   Includes bibliographical references and index.
   ISBN 0-87983-627-X : $16.95
   1. Nutrition. 2. Cookery (Natural foods) 3. Wheat-free diet—
Recipes. 4. Milk-free diet—Recipes. I. Title.
RA784.N68 1994
613.2—dc20   94-17631
                                             CIP

Printed in the United States of America

Published by Keats Publishing, Inc.
27 Pine Street (Box 876)
New Canaan, Connecticut 06840-0876

FOR ALL OF NATURE
SING WE OUR GRATEFUL PRAISE
TO THEE

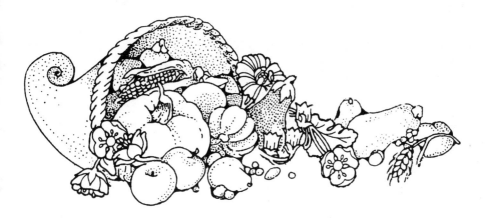

ACKNOWLEDGMENTS

My special thanks to those who first encouraged me to write
this book:

Charles C. Bell
Alan H. Nittler, M.D.
Leo Roy, M.D.

And to those who edited it and gave me their helpful critiques:

Sarah Bingham, M.A.
Michele Harrison, M.D.
Barbara Friedlander Meyer
Marshall Nostrand
Neil S. Orenstein, Ph.D.
Richard Roberts
Jairo Rodriguez, D.C.
Sproutman

To Floyd D. Page, who graciously offered me the use of his word
processor. Because of his generosity, patience and moral support,
the three years of typing and editing was a joy.

To Eva Graf, who has taught me much about nutritional cooking,
and who inspires me with the ease with which she creates delicious
and nutritious goodies.

To my clients, who kept asking me when this book would be
finished. It is their need that created it. I give it to them with love
and gratitude.

CONTENTS

Introduction

SECTION I

OVERCOMING CONFLICTS IN CHANGING YOUR DIET

1	*The Strange New World of Health Foods*	5
2	*Cost and Spoilage*	8
3	*Where to Shop*	9
4	*Getting to Know the Health Food Store*	10
5	*Preparation Time*	12
6	*Eating Out*	15
7	*Foods to Go for Work or Travel*	17
8	*Cooking for Others*	18
9	*Visiting Family and Friends*	21
10	*Food Cravings*	23

SECTION II

MAKING A SMOOTH TRANSITION
TO HEALTHIER FOODS

11	*Choosing Foods for Health*	29
12	*Avoiding Stressful Foods*	43
13	*Low Stress Change*	52
14	*Practical Tips for a Smooth Transition*	56
15	*Equipment & Utensils*	64
16	*Shopping Hints*	68
17	*Planning Your Meals*	71
18	*Protein in a Vegetarian Diet*	80
	Protein Combining Chart 81	

19   *Combining Foods for Better Digestion*   83
20   *Basic Food Preparation*   88

SECTION III
RECIPES

Important Notes   93
Tables   00
   Abbreviations of Measurements   94
   Weight and Metric Equivalents   94
   Liquid Volume Equivalents   95
   Common Food Equivalents   96
Sprouts   99
Breads & Muffins   108
Cereals   119
Pancakes   131
Eggs   135
Beverages   137
Soups   158
Salads   174
Dressing, Dips, Spreads & Sauces   184
Chicken   199
Fish   202
Vegetable Dishes   210
Grains   219
Pasta   237
Beans & Tofu   242
Snacks & Desserts   251

SECTION IV
APPENDIX

Natural Food Kitchen Hints   275
Hints for Easy Cleaning of Utensils   279
Common Food Additives   282
Hidden Sugar   286
Hidden Salt   288
Planned Menu Chart   290
Tips for Planned Menu Chart   291
Natural Foods Glossary   292

Index   303

INTRODUCTION

Why change your diet?

It may be because you are ill, and a dietary change has been recommended by your nutrition consultant or doctor.

Or, you have read that it can prevent illness later in life.

Or, perhaps you just don't feel as well as usual, and think that a better diet may help.

Or you wish to lose or gain weight.

Or a friend has changed his or her diet, and looks and feels much better.

Regardless of the reason, changing one's diet can present a confusing array of questions and conflicts.

We are used to eating certain foods. We know how to prepare them. We have our schedules and our lifestyles, and our diets fit into them. A change in diet often conjures up a threatening image of disruption and deprivation.

Your life does not need to be disrupted, and you do not need to be deprived of delicious goodies. With a few hints and guidelines and some easy, delicious recipes, a change in diet can be gradual, taking place with little stress. As the process unfolds, you will continuously be delighted with new taste treats which will more than replace your old favorites. As you make these discoveries, and find your own shortcuts, the process will become easier and more enjoyable.

Best of all, you will begin to experience increased health and vitality.

This book contains basic, practical information that can be helpful in making a transition to healthier foods, and delicious recipes that are highly nutritious and easy to prepare.

The book is divided into four sections.

The first section addresses the questions and conflicts most commonly faced when changing one's diet. The thought of these conflicts often prevents a change in diet, or can make a change more difficult. They are partially based on the *fear* of change, but they are real and important questions, and should be considered.

The second section of the book lists foods which support overall health, and those which do not, and contains practical methods for incorporating healthier foods into your life with ease.

This section also notes the types of foods necessary for a balanced diet, and how to combine them, and it contains lists, charts and other guidelines to help make a change with the least amount of stress.

The main portion, or third section, of the book contains recipes designed for great taste, simplicity in preparation, and maximum nutritional value. The foods used are vital foods—those which can aid any health maintenance or health regaining program. Many recipes are geared to one person, and can be easily multiplied. They are primarily milk- and wheat-free, since many people are allergic to wheat and milk.

Since this is a transition cookbook, I have included ingredients such as eggs, cheese and butter, which may not be part of your diet. Feel free to substitute an egg replacer (see page 61) or soy cheese or "better butter" (see page 36).

In addition to the recipes, simple cooking techniques with lists of variations are included in each recipe section. This helps eliminate elaborate planning ahead and assists you in experimenting with your own recipes. This gives you more flexibility to shop and plan meals according to your taste, nutritional requirements, financial situation, the climate and availability of fresh foods, and all the other variables that change from day to day.

The recipes are not limited to one particular type of diet, since we are all at varying stages of transition. There are recipes familiar to more "conventional" cooking, including chicken and fish, and there are recipes for diets which emphasize raw food, or grains and beans. In brief, recipes to be enjoyed by anyone who prefers great taste, good nutrition, and simplicity in preparation.

The fourth section of the book contains an appendix and an alphabetical index.

The appendix includes helpful reference material such as a "natural foods" glossary, natural foods kitchen hints, hints for cleaning utensils easily, a list of common food additives and their level of toxicity, and lists of "hidden" sugar and salt in processed foods. It also includes a planned menu chart for one week and tips for planning menus.

SECTION I

OVERCOMING CONFLICTS IN CHANGING YOUR DIET

Changing one's diet is an unfolding process of self-discovery, basically through trial and error, sometimes with the help of a nutrition consultant or doctor.

Profound and positive changes can take place mentally and emotionally, as well as physically, as your lifestyle and mental clarity are enhanced by the new, vital foods. Change, even when positive, is still a shock to the system, and sometimes small adjustments and compromises can help you adapt slowly until you are able to make more substantive changes when the time is right for you.

A change of diet should be gradual. That is, do not try to go from a "meat and potato" to a totally raw food diet unless advised and guided by your nutrition consultant or doctor to do so. Your body—physical, mental, emotional and spiritual—needs a chance to make necessary adjustments at its own pace.

Each step will evolve naturally from the last. This gives your system and your lifestyle time to adjust as you are ready. With a gradual transition you will also be less likely to become discouraged or bored with the new diet, and less likely to give it up, or to reject the changes it will make.

At the same time, exercise enough self-discipline to avoid the foods which contribute to ill health. This is crucial to keep the process moving toward better health. The more assiduously you avoid these foods, the more quickly you will lose your taste for them, and the more quickly your body will attain good health.

This section addresses the most common questions that arise when considering a change of diet. It helps to know that most of us are confronted with some of the same basic conflicts. Does this sound familiar?

- Will changing my diet really affect the quality of my health?
- What would it mean to my lifestyle? None of my friends eats that way. How could I go out to restaurants with them, or to their house for dinner? I don't want to be one of those fanatic health nuts who say they can't eat this or that.
- Is it really worth all the changes I have to make?
- Health foods are so expensive. How do you know that they're any better than the foods in my supermarket?
- I don't have time to plan and prepare foods. I have a really busy schedule, especially in the morning.
- What'll I do at work? There are no health food restaurants near me. Even if there were, they're too expensive to eat in every day. Could I take something with me to work? Like what?
- I'm too tired at the end of the day to prepare a meal. I need to grab something quick. I don't know how to cook health foods. Besides, I hate to cook.
- I know I should get a lot of variety in my diet, but I can't be bothered planning meals. It's so much easier eating the same foods over and over.
- I only cook for myself, and it's so boring to prepare a meal for one person.
- I cook for my family. They'll never eat this way, and I don't want to prepare different meals for everybody.
- I'm already depressed from not feeling well. Now, on top of

that, do I have to give up all my favorite foods? Are there really foods that are good for me that taste as good as my favorites?

These are all good questions. The answers aren't the same for everyone. Each of you will find your own solutions as you go through the process, but perhaps some of the discoveries my clients and I have made can be helpful.

One important common denominator for anyone changing their diet: a sense of humor. Don't be obsessive about the change. Find your own balance between being easy on yourself and pushing against your resistance to positive change. Keep the momentum going through self-discipline, self-respect, and self-love.

1

The Strange New World of Health Foods

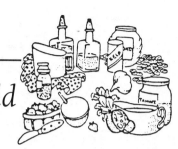

Eating "health food" does not mean taking away all the good things, and eating foods that are strange or boring, but good for you.

It means eating many of the same foods you love, but in a whole state, in the form Nature intended—what I call "real food": fresh fruits and vegetables, whole grains, beans, nuts and seeds, certain meat and dairy products and certain sweets. It may also mean simply changing your emphasis—eating less meat, dairy and sweets, and more fresh fruits and vegetables, whole grains, beans and nuts and seeds.

It means discovering the marvelous variety of delicious fruits and vegetables, including more of them in your diet, and preparing them with as little heat as possible, so that they retain their bright color, deep flavor, fiber, and nutrients.

It means enjoying your pasta and bread, while getting a health return from them, by eating them in a whole-grain state instead of a refined or processed state. With whole grains, the outer layer (or bran) and the inner core (or germ) of the grain has not been processed out, so you get fiber, B vitamins, vitamin E, protein and minerals along with a delicious nutty flavor that is absent in the processed grain.

The world of health foods may seem strange or new because some of these unprocessed foods are unfamiliar to you, but they certainly were not strange to our ancestors. They are foods which have supported life for generations.

Another reason eating healthy foods often seems strange is because it may mean changing some old habits. You may need to change the proportion of foods you eat—perhaps less red meat, less sweets, and more vegetables. You may need to find new stores, new ways of preparing foods, and different brands that are less processed and free of salt and sugar.

Once you have incorporated healthier foods into your daily routine and found your own short cuts, shopping and preparation will be easy. You'll find that it takes no more time to lightly steam fresh vegetables than to warm up frozen or canned vegetables, to make whole grain pasta or bread instead of refined. Even brown rice takes only half an hour, and the nutritional value in these unprocessed foods will give you additional health support.

Some of the foods within the range of "health foods" have come to us from other cultures. These foods can add health benefits and delicious taste variation to our recipes. They are not foods we were brought up on, so the taste, texture, preparation and association is not familiar to us. This is one of the strongest reasons we resist changing our diets and trying new foods. This is a very natural reaction.

For this reason, it is helpful to know something about any new food, and then to introduce it gradually by including it in familiar types of recipes. What was once unfamiliar may turn out to be one of your favorite foods!

Following are some of the foods included in this book which may be new to you. Refer to the glossary for more detailed information on each of these foods.

Agar agar: A jelling agent, like gelatin.

Arrowroot: A thickener used like cornstarch.

Carob: A bean, ground into a powder and used in place of chocolate.

Miso: Soy bean paste, used to add a deep, salty flavor to soups, sauces, etc.

Tahini: Sesame seed butter. It's something like peanut butter, but it's made with sesame seeds instead of peanuts.

Tamari: Soy sauce, used to add a deep, salty flavor and dark color to sauces, etc.

Tofu: Soy bean curd. Used in numerous ways as a protein, and in place of dairy.

Your recipes can be greatly enhanced by using different kinds of foods. Keep expanding, introducing new foods and new types of recipes. Allow yourself time to get to know the food, and to enjoy your discoveries.

2

Cost and Spoilage

In some cases, health foods cost more, simply because they spoil faster without the addition of toxic preservatives.

When you consider the cost of good food, take into account the quality of the foods, and the quality of health they reflect in your body. Good foods are an investment in your future—preventive "medicine."

Junk filler foods are also expensive. The sugar, salt and additives in them stimulate cravings for more, so you buy more. Eating more nutritious foods tends to satisfy longer than empty calorie foods, so that one is less likely to crave more. Healthy snacks, such as fresh or dried fruit, raw vegetables, nuts and seeds, though expensive, satisfy in smaller amounts and for a longer period of time.

If you have the storage space, certain foods such as whole grains and beans can be purchased in bulk to cut down on cost.

Naturally, with fresh foods and those with no preservatives there is greater chance for spoilage. This is especially a concern for small households. Fresh fruits and vegetables will need to be purchased more often, but sometimes they can be bought in smaller packages. If not, extra amounts need not go to waste. For example, leafy greens, such as lettuce or parsley, can be made into a delicious "green drink," and vegetables can be juiced.

In addition, there are many tips to help avoid spoilage. See "Natural Food Kitchen Hints" and "Shopping Hints."

Keep in mind that *good food tastes better!*

3

Where to Shop

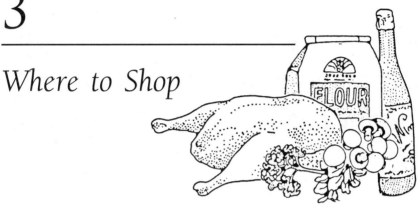

Most "health foods" are easily available, since fresh fruits and vegetables, some whole grains and beans and nuts and seeds can be purchased at your local market.

In discussing *quality* health foods and their availability, it is necessary to use a good-better-best guide. The highest quality health foods are the least processed—those closest to their natural state. In this case, the best source is your own farm, where you can pick organically grown fruits and vegetables fresh. Next best is a local organic farm, then a good health food store, food co-op or fruit and vegetable market.

If you are limited to shopping in a supermarket, read labels, become thoroughly aware of what you are buying, and demand the best quality. Find out when fruits and vegetables are delivered to the store and how long they have been on the truck, so that you can purchase them as fresh as possible.

Familiarize yourself with the most common toxic food additives, and with products that contain "hidden" sugar and salt. Refer to the appendix for lists of these additives and products. Take copies of these lists with you to the store.

If you cannot get the purest of foods, clean them as best you can (See "Kitchen Hints," pp. 275–281), then relax and enjoy them.

4

Getting to Know the Health Food Store

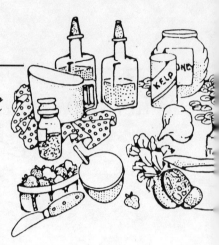

Most healthy foods—fresh fruits and vegetables, whole grains and beans—do not necessarily have to be purchased in a health food store. However, the health food store does contain good quality whole grains and beans, nuts and seeds, organic eggs and sometimes organic meats, farm-raised fish, fruits and vegetables, as well as un-processed, chemical- and sugar-free oils and condiments. (Organic meat and eggs are from animals raised free-range, fed with natural feed rather than chemicals, and not injected with hormones and antibiotics.) In addition, health food stores contain a wide variety of delicious ethnic foods such as tahini or miso.

Health food stores may feel intimidating at first—a maze of unfa-miliar foods, and a new language of nutrition, often associated with "health nuts" and faddism. Approach your health food store with an open mind. Try not to attach any negative associations to it, and don't be afraid of it. Consult friends, a nutritionist, and store clerks for the best brands to buy. Take along the list of staples on pp. 68–70 as a guide.

At first, just explore the health food store for the fun of it. Read labels, because not even everything in a health food store is healthy. Pick up a couple of items you would normally use—perhaps a delicious jam made with just fruit and no sugar or preservatives, a pure ice cream, a loaf of whole grain bread, or a box of whole grain, sugar-free cereal.

After you feel more comfortable, you may find yourself looking around more, noticing new foods. Read their labels. Ask about them and how they are used. It is a process of developing new relationships in your life. It will happen naturally, if you allow it. Eventually your health food store will be an old friend.

5

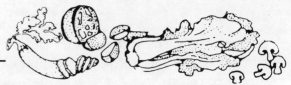

Preparation Time

Very few of us have time to spend hours planning and preparing a meal. In fact, many people find that they expend so much energy in their jobs and other daily activities that even the *thought* of planning a meal, looking up recipes, and shopping for specific ingredients causes stress, especially when the recipes and ingredients are unfamiliar.

There are several ways to make preparation easier:

A. Set up your kitchen so that the preparation flows more easily. Make sure you have good counter space, with a cutting board, and easy access to pots, utensils and spices that you use frequently. Give yourself the gift of basic equipment and utensils that will make your life easier.

B. Keep on hand some basic food staples that store well, and which can be used in a variety of ways to create whole meals.

C. Get to know the basic foods you need in a day to provide you with a balanced diet. This gives you an over-all format within which to work.

D. Learn a few basic, simple cooking techniques that are especially quick and easy, but which allow for variety, expansion and creativity. In this way you can be as simple or as elaborate as you have the time, energy or inspiration to be.

Knowing a few techniques eliminates the need for excessive planning ahead, for using recipes, or for shopping for specific ingredients. Instead, having a technical framework within which to work frees you to create recipes that fit your mood and/or nutritional needs, and to use foods which are fresh, already on hand, or easy to find.

Specific techniques, rather than specific recipes, also provide greater opportunity for variety, which is so important for a balanced diet.

Some examples of foods prepared with simple cooking techniques are blended soups, basic soups, blended cereals, nut milks, grain pilafs, quick blended sauces, quick steam soups or meals, meal-in-one sautés and easy salads. The recipe section includes a description of each technique, with lists of suggested ingredients, plus a few examples.

E. Become familiar with recipes that require very little time to plan or prepare, such as those in this book.

F. Although it is always best to prepare foods fresh (which is one of the advantages in using quick, basic cooking techniques), some foods store fairly well pre-prepared and kept in the refrigerator or freezer. Again, work with the "good, better, best guide." It's better to eat something prepared the night before than to grab junk food.

In deciding which foods to prepare ahead and store, choose those that store well and are versatile in their uses. This helps avoid boredom with eating the same food two or three days in a row. (Try not to eat foods beyond three days in a row, however. Variety is important for a balanced diet, and it is possible to manifest an allergic reaction to a food eaten too much, too often.

Here are some examples of foods which can be prepared ahead:

(1) Spreads, dressings or dips, such as miso-tahini spread (p. 193), tofu dip (p. 190), or tahini dip (p. 191). These keep well for several days stored in covered glass jars in the refrigerator. Add water to them to make sauces or dressings. See each recipe for their many uses.

(2). Sunburgers (p. 212) and lentil walnut burgers (p. 247) keep well in the freezer. They're good hot or cold as a snack, a meal, or to take to work.

(3) Brown rice or other grains. Cooked brown rice stores quite well (4 days in the refrigerator, 3 months in the freezer), and can be used in a variety of ways. Blend it with hot water as a cereal;

add it to soups; lightly sauté it by itself or with vegetables; put it into loaves, etc.

(4) Cooked beans can be kept in the freezer for three months or the refrigerator for three days. They can be added to vegetable soups or salads, made into burgers, or blended with hot water for a creamy bean soup, sauce or dip;

(5) Cooked chicken can be diced and added to cold salads, soups, vegetable dishes, made into curried chicken, etc.

(6) Sauerkraut can be eaten as is, added to salads, baked with potatoes, etc.

(7) Leafy greens, such as lettuce, parsley, watercress, or Swiss chard, can be washed, cut up and kept in a plastic lettuce container. They are then ready to add to salads, vegetable loaves or green drinks.

(8) Raw vegetables can be washed, chopped and refrigerated, ready to add to salads, soups, vegetable dishes, juices, or as snacks with dips.

Please note that washing or slicing vegetables and greens ahead of time results in extreme loss of nutrients, so in general it is not advised. Again, use the "good-better-best" guide.

As you become familiar with the cooking techniques, with "new" foods, and with the recipes in this book, food preparation will become easier and take less time. You will begin to find ways of making your own adjustments and shortcuts. It is a process of learning and discovery. Take your time, incorporating new techniques as you are ready. Enjoy it well!

6

Eating Out

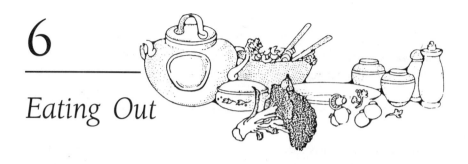

Usually, we associate eating out with relaxing, enjoying ourselves, and eating what most appeals to us on the menu. The foods with appeal are sometimes those that do not support over-all health and vitality—those that are "creamy, gooey, fatty or fried." We need to change our associations, and break our habits of choosing foods which put stress on our bodies and our health. We usually choose the same restaurants, and the same foods on the menu. Begin to look at menus with a different eye, and you will see that there really are healthful foods you can choose.

Appetizers are often foods you can enjoy, such as freshly made soups, poached salmon, artichokes, salads, or steamed or grilled vegetables. Some people enjoy a meal of just appetizers.

For an entrée, most restaurants offer fresh fish, lamb, baked chicken or other fowl as well as lightly steamed vegetables, baked potatoes and salads, and sometimes whole grains.

When choosing from entrées, avoid dishes that are high in fat, or are overly cooked, fried (such as tempura or fried chicken), heavily salted or sugared, or drenched in rich sauces or thick, gooey cheese. In some restaurants, it is possible to ask that the sauce be put on the side, or that the food be cooked without fat. Many restaurants are now accustomed to such requests and are willing to fulfill them.

It may also be wise to avoid pork or shellfish, which are often contaminated.

Usually desserts are the worst offender in restaurants. Order fresh

15

fruit, have your dessert at home, or "restaurant hop." Have your dessert at a health food restaurant, where you can order a dessert made without processed flour or sugar. Restaurant hopping also gives you time to digest your main course before having your dessert.

If you eat at more expensive restaurants, you are more likely to get fresh, good quality food, low in fat and not over-cooked. To cut down on the cost of a better restaurant, avoid the non-foods which put additional stress on the body and limit the digestion of your meal—excessive alcohol, sugary desserts, coffee, teas containing caffeine or tannin.

Don't stuff yourself. Light eating is easier on the digestion as well as the pocket book. If the portions are more than you can eat, take the rest home! You'll get two or three meals for the price of one.

Sometimes it helps to eat a snack at home before you go to a restaurant. This may sound silly, but it serves several purposes:

1. When you are less hungry, your will power is stronger. You are less likely to order and eat more food than your body can digest.

2. By ordering less, you'll spend less, yet still have the pleasure of dining out with friends.

3. By spending less, you can choose a finer restaurant with better quality food and more pleasant atmosphere.

4. If you are with friends who do not eat as you do, and you go to a restaurant which has a limited menu, you won't mind eating less. Usually a delicious appetizer and one or two special side dishes are plenty to eat and nutritionally perfect.

5. When you are less famished, and your will power is greater, you are more likely to order foods which are right for you to eat rather than the less nutritious foods with an "emotional pull."

Good foods to eat before you go out are: baked squash, baked potato, raw vegetables with a dip, artichoke, soup, yogurt or fruit.

Eating out is usually a festive occasion, a time for being with friends. Eating well can only add to your enjoyment.

7

Foods To Go For Work Or Travel

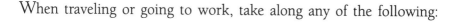

When traveling or going to work, take along any of the following:

nuts and seeds
soaked dried fruit
fresh fruit and vegetables
pure juices
soups in a thermos, or soup bouillon cubes or powders to be
    mixed with hot water
herb tea bags
whole-grain breads and crackers
homemade granola or granola bought in a health food store

Snacks can be carried in small plastic bags and/or small plastic containers, wide-mouthed thermos bottles, Mason jars, etc. Canvas carrying bags with a shoulder strap, lined with washable, water-resistant fabric or plastic, can be purchased or made.

Sometimes left-overs can be used, or quick foods can be prepared in the morning.

When traveling, stopping at a roadside restaurant is a welcome break, and yet the menu is often less than desirable. If you have munched on good snacks along the way, at least you won't be so hungry that you'll feel the need to order something you may regret later. Most roadside restaurants have soups, and many have salad bars which range from adequate to excellent.

17

8

Cooking for Others

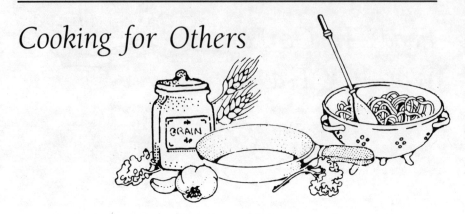

Cooking for family and friends can present a whole new set of challenges.

At the same time, it gives you the opportunity to introduce your family to more delicious recipes, and gives you the pleasure of feeding them foods which support their good health.

Usually, if you just prepare what you love, it will be a huge success with everyone. (Warning: Don't tell them you are feeding them "health food." Just tell them it's a new recipe you are trying.)

In some cases, it may be better at first to use familiar recipes they enjoy, but with healthy changes. Following are a few ideas which will be discussed and illustrated more fully in Section II.

A. Convert recipes, substituting healthful ingredients for stressful ones. For example, use whole grain flour in place of white flour. Use honey in place of sugar. Use brown rice in place of white rice.

Sometimes the conversion can take place gradually. For example, at first use a combination of whole grain flour with white flour or brown rice with white rice, or whole grain noodles with processed noodles. Increase the proportion of whole grain to processed as you and your family are ready.

B. Supplement recipes, adding nutritious ingredients to your present recipes.

18

C. Use recipes that are the same types of foods as those your family enjoys. For example, make sunburgers instead of hamburgers, and use a sugar- and chemical-free ketchup on top. Make cookies and candies out of whole grains, nuts and seeds, honey and dried fruit instead of white flour and sugar.

Other good recipes for family and guests who are accustomed to traditional American cuisine are the following (see Recipes section):

Appetizers: mixed raw vegetables with spring green dip, vegetable soup, potato leek soup, artichokes.

Main Course: coq au vin, any of the fish recipes, wild rice casserole.

Dessert: zucchini bread, fresh fruit ice cream, strawberries with carob sauce.

D. Explore the health food store and purchase products which resemble those your family enjoys. For example, there are delicious whole grain cereals, breads and condiments such as jellies, mayonnaise and ketchup that are made without sugar or toxic additives. There are ice cream and soft drinks made without sugar—even beer made without alcohol.

E. When cooking for children, have them share in the preparation. Children usually enjoy helping prepare meals when it is treated as something fun you are doing together, rather than a chore. And, they appreciate the food more.

Teach them how to grow sprouts. Children love to grow sprouts, and usually love to eat them. Include sprouts as much as possible in their meals, particularly if they don't enjoy salads.

Children are more likely to eat raw vegetables if given to them in small pieces to munch on, with a dip. Blend cottage cheese and herbs in a blender or use any of the recipes in this book. Or, use almond butter purchased in a health food store, or made at home.

Another way to give children vegetables is in the form of fresh juices.

At party time, or whenever you feel inspired, you can arrange chopped vegetables or fruits in designs and funny faces. For example, cherry tomatoes for eyes, 1/2 sliced green pepper for ears, sliced mushrooms for a nose, a slice of beet for a mouth with corn for teeth, and celery leaves or parsley for hair.

There are many desserts and snacks that your children will love, which will nourish them at the same time, such as fresh fruit ice cream, nut/seed candies, etc.

Make any changes gradually. Don't worry; your family and friends will love the new recipes. They are delicious, and your guests will feel better eating them.

9

Visiting Family and Friends

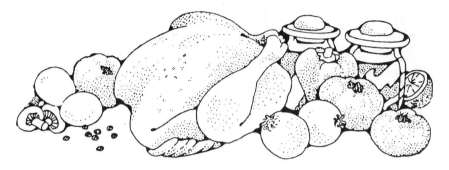

From time to time you may be the object of some teasing. This is especially difficult with family, since loved ones may feel that your new diet is a rejection of them, and an attack on your upbringing. You have to decide how much you can share about your new understandings and how much you can compromise in eating with them. Tension created in certain situations can create more stress in your body than any foods.

If you decide it is best to share their meal, relax and enjoy it, fully digest the love that went into preparing it for you, and enjoy the company!

There are times when you can offer to prepare a meal for others. This is a good opportunity to introduce them to your new way of eating, but use recipes that are not too different from theirs. Remember that your way is not necessarily right for them.

You could also bring something with you for dessert or a snack. A few examples of house gifts are "sunny snack," p. 252; oatmeal cookies, p. 258; a pure honey vanilla ice cream with a jar of carob mint sauce, p. 272; zucchini bread, p.113, or gingered carrot marmalade, p. 197. You could package the gifts with ribbons, attractive labels, dried or fresh flowers, etc.

If you decide not to eat with family or friends, try not to explain too much, as it usually complicates matters. You can always say that you have discovered that certain foods do not agree with you, or that your doctor or nutritionist has you on a restricted diet. Usually, the less you say, the better.

The most difficult times will be when you yourself doubt the validity of your new regime. Most people go through periods when, as their bodies release toxins, they experience discomfort. If you are not sure what this discomfort is, check with your nutrition consultant or doctor, and don't give up. The crisis will pass and you will be stronger in mind and body than before.

Eventually your family and friends will get used to your new way of eating. Just love them, and let them know you are not judging their diet. They will eventually accept the new healthier you.

10

Food Cravings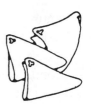

Food cravings can indicate many things.

They can mean your body lacks nutrients. If you eat nutrient-poor foods, your body will continuously send out signals for more food until it is satisfied. Eating nutrient-rich foods, therefore, can help prevent cravings.

Cravings for sweet or salty foods can indicate a blood sugar imbalance, which can result from excesses of sugar or nutrient-poor foods, stress, emotional trauma, inherent weakness, etc. In this case, it would probably be best to avoid all sweets, including honey, molasses, maple syrup, fruit juices and dried fruit, until the blood sugar imbalance is corrected. Otherwise, even these natural sweets can trigger a sugar binge similar to an alcoholic's craving for alcohol. This situation, which is quite common, should be under the care of a nutrition consultant or doctor.

Cravings for sweet foods can also be stimulated by consuming an excess of salty foods, and vice versa. This is the body's attempt to balance these excesses. Moderation in eating such foods is important.

Cravings can be clues to food sensitivities. Sometimes we crave the very foods to which we are allergic. This can apply even to healthy foods like whole wheat bread, corn, or eggs. Eating the allergen stops the craving and gives you an initial high. Unfortunately, it results in a let-down later and contributes to further breakdown of the body. It is similiar to an alcoholic addiction. The craving is stimulated by withdrawal symptoms which are postponed

23

by eating the food. It usually takes five days for the craving to subside.

Food cravings can be the result of dehydration. Sometimes we eat foods when we are actually thirsty. Very often, people who are overweight find that drinking more water (and eating nutrient-rich foods) helps reduce their desire for food.

Food cravings can also be from lack of oxygen in the body, and from blocked, frustrated creative energy. Deep breathing, and finding positive outlets for your creativity can help.

There is a great deal of emotional attachment to food, as well. This is a subject for an entire book. To touch on it briefly, however, there is, for example, often a connection between sugar and reward, love or approval. Food becomes a substitute for love and nourishment on a deep level. The pain of the emotions connected with the lack of love, including self-love and a spiritual awareness, is suppressed by eating. Examine your attachments to food closely. If you can avoid the desired food, yet allow yourself to experience the emotions surrounding it, you can learn a great deal about yourself, and help release the need for the food.

You will find that as you eliminate one undesirable food from your diet, you will lose your appreciation for another that you thought would be difficult to give up. As the body cleanses itself of toxic matter, it becomes more sensitive to the taste and effect of food. Devitalized food will taste dead, sugar will seem too sweet, coffee will have too strong an effect, etc.

Remember the "good, better, best" guide. Find a "good" substitute for the food you crave and eat that for a while. Then substitute a "better" food, and eventually eat the "best" foods.

For example, substitute a carob bar (without sugar) for chocolate. After a short time, switch to home-made carob candies, since many of the store-bought carob bars contain oils which are difficult to digest. Then, eat fruit instead of candies.

Another example: substitute water-processed decaffeinated coffee for regular coffee. After a short time switch to pure grain beverages, such as Pero or Cafix, and to herb teas.

Another example: have a sugar-free ice cream in place of ice cream with sugar or chemicals. Then switch to ice creams made from fresh fruit without dairy.

If you have a craving for a food that seems healthy to you, try it and note your reaction. It could be something you lack and you will feel better eating it—not just right away, but for hours afterward.

Discuss your cravings with your nutrition consultant or physician. Eventually you will be able to distinguish between what is a craving for an allergen and what you are actually lacking.

If you give in to a craving and eat something you are trying to give up, examine how you felt before and after. Record any negative reactions you had (but don't expect them), then resolve to be stronger next time. Each time it will be easier to exercise more self control. As your body becomes less toxic, the cravings will become less and less and finally will fall away.

SECTION II:

MAKING A SMOOTH TRANSITION TO HEALTHIER FOODS

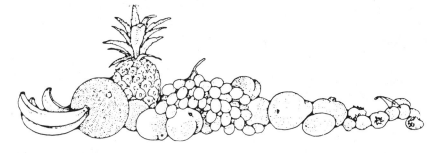

Our bodies are constantly striving for health. Any health-regaining program has the same basic principle:

Rebuilding the weak organs and tissues and replenishing the body with all needed essential proteins, vitamins, minerals, oils and enzymes; and detoxifying the body, or getting rid of toxic waste that has caused an imbalance, or has prevented the body from functioning to its fullest capacity.

Food is a vital and very basic part of any health-regaining program since, ideally, it helps regenerate our body structures through its nourishing properties, and aids in the elimination of toxic matter.

There are certain foods which generally support the life-giving process, and there are certain foods which inhibit this process, causing further stress and contributing to physical and mental breakdown.

In general, the foods you choose should be as close to their natural state as possible. They should be whole, unprocessed, and without toxic additives. The closer foods are to the state in which they grew, the more vitality they contain and will transfer to you.

Meal planning, preparation and consumption of foods should be geared toward maximum preservation and assimilation of nutrients as well as great taste.

Each of us has special needs, both nutritional and practical, which affect the foods we choose and the ways in which we plan and prepare our meals. For everyone, good taste, simplicity in preparation and a diet that is healthy and fits into one's life style is essential.

A change of diet must, therefore, be as smooth, as delicious and as easily workable as possible while still maintaining good nutrition.

This section will present guidelines which can be helpful in making a smooth transition to a better diet geared to individual needs. The following points will be considered:

- Foods which generally support good health, and those which lead to ill health (Chapters 11 and 12).

- How to change without stress (Chapters 13–14).

- How to make a diet practical and easy without sacrificing good taste and nutrition (Chapters 15–20).

11

Choosing Foods For Health

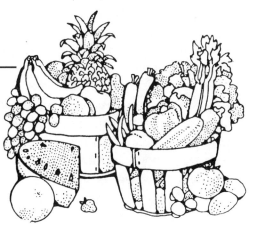

The foods which most support over-all health are whole grains, nuts and seeds, sprouts, beans and peas, fresh fruits and vegetables, eggs, certain meat, fish and dairy products, certain oils, sweeteners and seasonings, fresh fruit and vegetable juices, herb teas, and pure water.

All of these foods will be most delicious and nutritious if they are as unadulterated, as fresh and as whole as possible.

FOODS TO ENJOY

WHOLE GRAINS

whole wheat	brown rice	barley
cornmeal	millet	rye
bulgur (cracked wheat)	oats	amaranth
buckwheat and kasha (buckwheat groats)		quinoa

Grains can be either whole or refined.

A refined grain is one that has been altered in processing. Manufacturers remove the outer layer and the inner core of the grain for two reasons: first, the inner core of the grain (the germ) spoils and is the nutritious part bugs like to eat. Removing the germ will extend the shelf life of the grain, yielding higher profits. Secondly, removing the germ along with the outer layer, or bran, will make the grain white and lighter in texture, satisfying consumer preference.

A whole grain has the germ and the bran intact. The germ contains most of the important essential nutrients in the grain. For example, whole wheat contains 50 to 80 percent more nutrients than white flour, including B vitamins, vitamin E, phosphorus, iron, zinc, copper, magnesium and chromium. The bran, which acts as fiber, helps prevent constipation and chronic diseases such as heart disease, cancer and diabetes. A refined grain such as white flour gives us mostly starch and calories without the nutritional benefits. Whole grains also have a delicious, nutty flavor that is absent in refined grains and the fiber content helps fill us up so that we are less likely to overeat.

The most common grain that is used is wheat, and most of it is refined. Refined wheat flour is what we call white flour, the flour used to make most breads, cakes, cookies and pasta. However, whole wheat breads, pasta and other flour products are now widely available in supermarkets as well as health food stores. If the ingredients on the label read "made with wheat," it is probably refined wheat, or white flour. The label must read "whole grain" or "whole wheat" to specify unrefined. Besides white flour and whole wheat flour, couscous and bulgur are other forms of wheat.

Wheat is only one of many grains. Other grains include rice (brown rice is whole grain rice; white rice is refined), cornmeal, barley, oats, millet, buckwheat and kasha (roasted buckwheat) rye, kamut, spelt, teff, and the recently rediscovered grains amaranth and quinoa. It is best to eat a variety of grains especially because wheat is a common allergen, and over-eating wheat products can stimulate the allergic response. Many breads, cereals and pastas in the health food store are wheat-free.

SPROUTS

Sprouts can be grown from nuts, seeds, grains or beans. The most common sprouts are:

alfalfa	buckwheat	lentil
sunflower	mung	chia
pumpkin	wheat	oat
rye	fenugreek	radish

Sprouts are good sources of protein, vitamins, minerals and fiber. Sunflower and buckwheat sprouts, in particular, are delicious in salads and sandwiches and may be eaten raw. Other sprouts should be cooked in order to remove naturally occurring toxins.

BEANS AND PEAS (LEGUMES)

aduki	kidney	mung
garbanzo	lentil	soy
split peas	pinto	black
navy beans		

Beans and peas are excellent sources of protein, especially when combined with grains, nuts and seeds or dairy, and, unlike meat or dairy, they are free of saturated fat and cholesterol. In addition, they are high in soluble fiber, the type of fiber that lowers cholesterol, promotes healthy elimination and may prevent or ease cancer and diabetes. They also contain iron, magnesium, zinc and B vitamins. The absorption of iron in beans is enhanced when eaten with foods high in vitamin C, such as tomatoes, potatoes or peppers.

NUTS AND SEEDS

flax seeds	sesame seeds	almonds
pumpkin seeds	sunflower seeds	walnuts
pecans	brazil nuts	filberts
chestnuts	chia seeds (seeds of the sage brush, high in protein)	

These are the best of nuts and seeds. I excluded peanuts, actually a legume, because they are a common allergen and often contain a mold which has been found to be cancer-causing. I also excluded cashews since they have a caustic oil, and macadamia nuts, which are higher in fat than any other nut (95% fat).

Nuts and seeds, nut butters and nut milks are all high in fat and therefore calories, but it is mostly unsaturated fat, the kind that doesn't clog arteries. Almonds and walnuts, in particular, contain monounsaturated fat, a kind of fat that may benefit the heart. Of course, nuts and seeds have no cholesterol, which is found only in animal products. They are rich in fiber and contain protein, vitamins B and E and minerals such as calcium, iron, potassium, zinc and magnesium.

When you purchase nuts, select those without added salt, honey or preservatives. Roasted nuts are usually fried in coconut oil, a highly saturated oil.

As with all oil-rich foods, nuts and seeds become rancid easily in processing, such as grinding, or when removed from their shells and exposed to warm temperatures. Ideally, it is best to purchase nuts and seeds in their shell and eat them right away or refrigerate them. Otherwise, be sure they are as fresh as possible or vacuum-packed. Rancid nuts have a bitter after-taste and are often soft, whereas fresh nuts have a sweet after-taste. If you grind your nuts and seeds ahead of time, keep them in a jar in the freezer and use them as soon as possible.

EGGS

Eggs are an excellent source of protein (divided equally between the white and the yolk), vitamins A, D, B12, E, folic acid and panto-thenic acid and the minerals iron, selenium, phosphorus, zinc, and sulfur.

Many people are concerned about eating egg yolks since three-fourths of the egg's calories and all of the cholesterol are in the yolk. For most individuals the cholesterol in the egg is not harmful, however, and since the yolk provides most of the essential nutrients, it should not be eliminated from one's diet unless recommended by a health professional. The American Heart Association suggests that healthy individuals eat a maximum of four eggs per week. In many recipes, two egg whites can be used in place of one whole egg and in recipes that call for two eggs, use one whole egg and two whites. (Note, however, that the egg white is a common allergen.)

Some studies have shown that the method of cooking an egg influences the effect of cholesterol on the heart. Eggs cooked with high heat, as in frying or hard boiling, produce the highest levels of blood cholesterol, whereas soft boiling or poaching an egg pro-duce the least effect. Unfortunately undercooking raises the potential of bacteria poisoning. The recommended cooking time to destroy bacteria is seven minutes for boiling, five minutes for poaching and three minutes on each side for frying.

I recommend using organic eggs rather than non-organic. Organic eggs are free of toxic by-products found in non-organic eggs such as antibiotics, hormones and pesticides. In general, organic eggs are also less likely to be contaminated with salmonella bacteria due to a stronger shell that keeps bacteria out, a healthier hen that is more resistent to disease, and cleaner growing conditions. Organic eggs taste better, have a darker yolk and firmer white and may have nutritional advantages as well, since they are laid by hens fed from roasted whole grains.

FISH

Fish is an excellent source of protein, B vitamins, iodine, phosphorus, selenium and other trace minerals. It is also relatively low in cholesterol and low in saturated fat, yet high in the types of oil (vitamin E and Omega-3 fatty acids) that may reduce the risk of heart disease and help alleviate or prevent rheumatoid arthritis, psoriasis, allergies and many other health problems. Fatty fish in particular, such as tuna, mackerel, salmon, shad, sardines, herring and bluefish, are high in these beneficial oils. They are also higher in fat calories, however, so you may want to alternate them with lower-fat fish such as haddock, sole, flounder or cod.

Recently there has been some concern over eating fish due to the possibility of contamination by bacteria or viruses or by toxic metals, pesticides and waste from polluted waters.

To avoid bacterial contamination, be sure the fish is fresh. The flesh should feel moist, firm and slightly springy to the touch. The gills should be reddish in color. The eyes should be bright and clear. It should smell sea-water fresh. Make sure it is refrigerated well, including at the market.

To avoid toxic metals such as lead and mercury, pesticides and chlorinated hydrocarbons like PCB's, DDT and dioxin, eat ocean fish or freshwater fish from mountain streams or hatcheries. In general, the safer fish are mackerel, cod, haddock, pollack, salmon, yellowfin tuna, flounder, perch, freshwater bass, brook or rainbow trout. Farm-raised fish are also generally less contaminated, but the inspection laws are inadequate.

When selecting fish, choose young, small fish which have had less time to accumulate contaminants. Trim away the internal organs and fatty parts of the fish such as the skin, dark meat and the fatty tissues along the back, sides and belly since those parts of the fish concentrate the contaminants.

In general it is best to avoid raw fish and shellfish (mussels, clams, oysters) since they may contain worms, parasites, bacteria, viruses and other contaminants. People with compromised immune function and pregnant and lactating women in particular should avoid raw fish and shellfish and fish that are more likely to be contaminated with mercury, hydrocarbons and other toxic chemicals, such as swordfish, carp, catfish, lake trout, whitefish, bluefish, eel and striped bass. In addition, some doctors recommend that pregnant and lactating women eat no more than half a pound per week of tuna, halibut, bass, swordfish, turbot, perch, pike or sheepshead, since these fish may be contaminated with mercury.

This sounds like an essay on Foods to Avoid, rather than Foods to Enjoy, but remember there are still lots of good fish to eat, and fish contains vital nutrients that will help your body resist any of the negative effects of contaminants.

MEAT AND POULTRY

Meat and poultry are rich sources of protein, iron, zinc and B vitamins. In fact, few foods are as rich in these nutrients as meat and poultry. However, meat in particular is high in saturated fat and cholesterol. Saturated fat contributes twice as much cholesterol to the blood as does cholesterol in foods.

The leanest beef is select eye of round or select top round; the leanest veal is leg or sirloin: the leanest pork is tenderloin or center loin. Select organic meats whenever possible.

Lamb, although still high in fat, contains fewer antibiotics and hormones than other red meats and is easier to digest. For those who prefer not to eliminate red meat, lamb is a good transition food. The leanest cuts of lamb are from the leg and loin.

White meat skinned chicken and turkey have 20 percent less saturated fat than red meat. When possible, use organically raised chicken since it will be free of hormones, antibiotics and other chemicals. Organic poultry is also more tender and delicious and generally less fatty. Skin the chicken after cooking to retain the moisture; the fat from the skin will not migrate to the meat.

DAIRY

goat's milk, goat cheese and goat yogurt
unsalted butter
plain non-fat yogurt
kefir drink (liquefied yogurt)
cheeses that break easily such as cottage, feta, pot, goat, farmer's

Cow's milk is a common allergen and unless labelled skim or low fat, is high in saturated fat. The above dairy products are high in calcium and seem to be digested and assimilated better than cow's milk itself.

Use unsalted butter in moderation. To make butter healthier, mix it with an equal amount of olive, flaxseed or canola oil. Beat oil into softened butter until you have a spreadable consistency. Store in the refrigerator. Some call this mixture "better butter;" my husband calls it simply "better."

OILS

olive oil
canola oil
cold pressed sesame, sunflower, flaxseed, soy, almond, avocado
   and walnut oil
unsalted butter (raw, if possible)

Cold pressed oils are those which have been extracted from the nut, seed or bean with low heat and with no chemicals, bleaching or deodorizing. They can be purchased in health food stores. The label will read "cold pressed."

Oils should be refrigerated to avoid rancidity. If you rarely use them, store them in the freezer, refrigerating a small amount.

Adding 200–400 I.U. of vitamin E to your oils can help protect them against oxidation which leads to rancidity.

When cooking with oils, use very low heat and use olive oil, canola oil or butter, since they will not break down and become toxic on high heats as easily as other oils. Never heat flaxseed oil.

For some people, soy oil on an ongoing basis can be congesting, since it is a common allergen. Vary it with other oils.

Vary your oils as much as possible to get a fuller range of essential fatty acids and nutrients.

BEVERAGES

> water
> nut milk or grain water
> pure fruit or vegetable juice
> certified raw cow's milk or goat's milk

Drink six to eight glasses of water a day. Preferably use spring water, or (if recommended by your nutrition consultant or doctor), distilled water.

VEGETABLES

Vegetables are good sources of vitamins, such as beta-carotene (or provitamin A), C and B; of minerals, such as potassium, magnesium, iron and calcium; of amino acids and water. Raw vegetables are one of our best sources of fiber.

The leafy greens are especially high in vitamins C, beta-carotene and B, in iron and calcium, and in chlorophyll, which is an important blood-builder. Include them in your diet daily.

Sea vegetables, or sea weeds, are extremely rich in minerals, especially iodine. They can be purchased dried in a whole or powdered form. You may need to become accustomed to their sea-weed flavor and association, but once you have, they can be an important adjunct to a nutritionally sound and tasty diet. Try adding them to soups at first.

FRUITS

Fruits are a good source of vitamins, especially beta-carotene and vitamin C, minerals, natural sugars, fiber, and water.

Fresh fruits should be eaten ripe, since their simple sugars are then more easily digested and assimilated. Try to use fruits that are in season.

Dried fruits contain concentrated fruit sugar, fiber, minerals, and some vitamins. Be sure your dried fruits are unsulfured, which means that the toxic chemical sulfur dioxide has not been added.

Please note that dried fruits are high in sugar and should be moderated or avoided by those with blood sugar problems. For many people, oranges and grapefruit are too acidic, and should be limited.

SWEETENERS

raw honey
unsulfured molasses
rice bran syrup
unsweetened carob powder
unsulfured dried fruit

barley malt
pure maple syrup
pure fruit juices

A note on honey vs. sugar: Although the body reacts to honey as sugar, raw honey has some nutrients and antibiotic properties that sugar does not have. Therefore, honey gives the body something in return, while sugar does nothing but cause depletion and stress.

Molasses and maple syrup, although "natural" sugars, are extremely concentrated. Molasses also has small amounts of calcium and iron; barley malt has small amounts of B vitamins.

Don't over-do your use of any of these natural sweeteners. It's especially easy to over-eat dried fruit, which in addition to being high in calories, sticks to your teeth, contributing to tooth decay.

SEASONINGS

cayenne pepper (add after cooking to preserve the vitamin C
and niacin.)

sea salt contains 75% sodium as well as other minerals, and is
therefore more balanced and less stressful than common table
salt, which is pure sodium chloride. However, limit all salts.

gomasio (sea salt and roasted sesame seeds)

soy sauce

apple cider vinegar (unpasteurized, if possible)

pure vanilla, orange or almond extract

dried vegetable powders and powdered dulse or kelp, which are
powdered seaweeds

herbs and spices:

allspice	comfrey	mustard	dill
oregano	caraway	nutmeg	basil
bay leaves	parsley	oregano	sage
coriander	garlic	cloves	mint
chili powder	cinnamon	ginger	thyme
tarragon	marjoram	chives	cumin

VEGETABLES

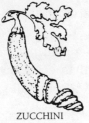

ZUCCHINI

ARTICHOKE

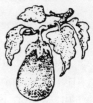

EGGPLANT

JERUSALEM ARTICHOKE
(SUNCHOKE)

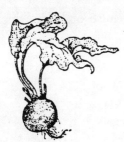

BEET

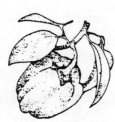

GREEN OR RED PEPPER

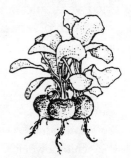

RADISHES

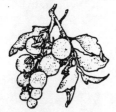

CHERRY TOMATOES*

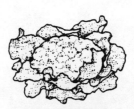

CAULIFLOWER

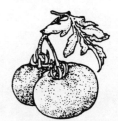

TOMATOES*

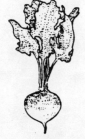

TURNIP

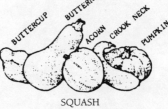

BUTTERCUP BUTTERNUT ACORN CROOK NECK PUMPKIN

SQUASH

PARSNIP

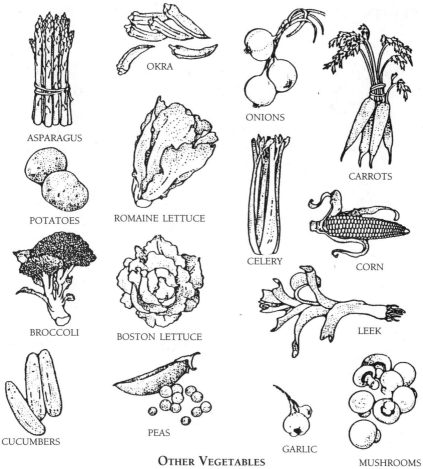

ASPARAGUS

OKRA

ONIONS

CARROTS

POTATOES

ROMAINE LETTUCE

CELERY

CORN

BROCCOLI

BOSTON LETTUCE

LEEK

CUCUMBERS

PEAS

GARLIC

MUSHROOMS

OTHER VEGETABLES

red cabbage	yam	snow peas	waterchestnut
white cabbage	sweet potato	lima beans	green string bean
chinese cabbage	daikon radish	scallions	yellow string bean

LEAFY GREENS

watercress, parsley, basil, mint, carrot tops, beet greens, turnip greens, dandelion greens, mustard greens, kale, Swiss chard, spinach, sorrel, endive, comfrey, escarole, chicory, arugula

EDIBLE SEA VEGETABLES

kombu, hijiki, dulse, arame, wakame, kanten, kelp

*Note: Although tomatoes are actually a fruit, they are usually eaten as if a vegetable.

FRUITS

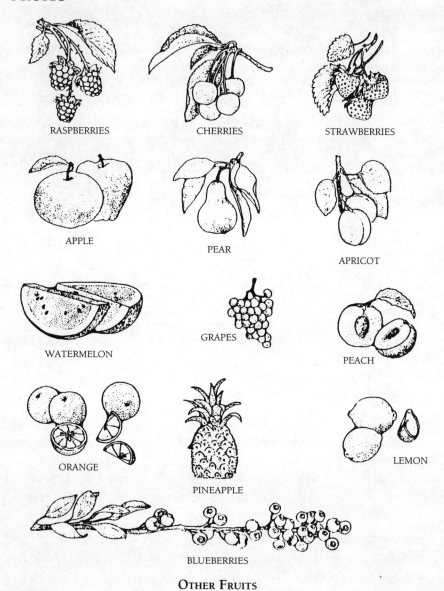

RASPBERRIES

CHERRIES

STRAWBERRIES

APPLE

PEAR

APRICOT

WATERMELON

GRAPES

PEACH

ORANGE

PINEAPPLE

LEMON

BLUEBERRIES

Other Fruits

| papaya | mango | raisin | prune | kiwi |
| banana | currant | fig | persimmon | avocado |

12

Avoiding Stressful Foods

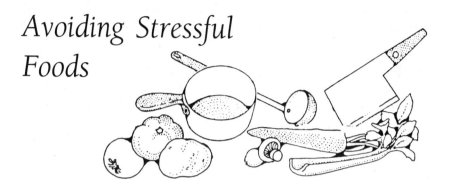

Foods which contribute to mental and physical deterioration are those foods which are farthest from their natural state. They have been processed, refined, adulterated with chemicals, sugar or salt, over-cooked, fried, or are rancid.

Processed foods harm the body in several ways:

(1) They have no nutrients so they give nothing to the body; or,

(2) They are toxic or stressful, because of their additives, or manner of processing or cooking.

(3) They demand energy and nutrients from other foods to digest and assimilate;

(4) They fill you up, replacing foods which do nourish you. This is one reason junk foods cause weight gain and imbalance of the entire metabolism.

(5) Because of the above reasons, they contribute to chronic disease, such as diabetes, heart disease, etc.

Learn to read labels. Keep in your pocket a list of the most common food additives and their level of toxicity. Not all additives are toxic. For a guide in distinguishing between which are toxic and which are not, refer to the appendix for a list of additives most commonly used in packaged foods.

In addition to toxic additives, processed foods are heavily dosed with sugar or salt. Americans consume more than 13 tablespoons of sugar *per day,* and 10 times more salt than is needed. The major portion of the sugar and salt consumed is in processed foods, not from the sugar bowl or salt shaker. If you feel you eat very little salt or sugar, but still eat processed foods, read labels, and refer to the lists of hidden sugars and hidden salt in foods, pp. 286 and 288. You may be in for a surprise.

Keep in mind that ingredients are listed in order of weight—the highest amount listed first. For example, if sugar is listed first, there is more sugar than any other ingredient. Also remember that there are many types of sugar.

In many cases the ingredients do not have to be listed and there are hidden sugars and other chemicals. Whenever possible, use fresh foods rather than packaged.

Choose only the best and purest foods. If you refuse to buy processed foods, there will eventually be a change in the market place. It's an investment in your good health, and you deserve it!

STRESSFUL FOODS TO AVOID

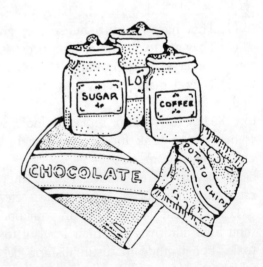

FOODS LACED WITH SUGAR

Sugar has many names. White sugar, brown, turbinado (which is white sugar with molasses added), glucose, fructose, sucrose, corn syrup, sorbitol, mannitol, malitol, xylitol and dextrose—all are refined sweeteners devoid of nutritional value, taking away from precious reserves of energy while giving nothing in return.

Sugar contributes to tooth decay and gum disease, and can aggravate blood sugar problems such as hypoglycemia, diabetes, overeating, arthritis, alcoholism, drug addiction, schizophrenia, nervous and behavioral disorders, and yeast problems. Sugar in all of its forms including fructose may also elevate the concentration of triglycerides and LDL cholesterol in the blood, encouraging heart disease, and, although testing is not conclusive, it may stress the immune system, making the body more susceptible to disease. Sorbitol and mannitol may cause diarrhea, gas and bloating, especially in young children.

Artificial sweeteners are equally harmful and may be even worse than refined sugar since they are chemicals with unknown effects on the body. Saccharin, acesulfame K (Sweet One and Sunette) and cyclamate (Sweet 'n Low) may increase the risk of cancer. Aspartame (Equal and NutraSweet) may cause headaches, dizziness, menstrual problems, increased risk for cancer or allergic reactions such as hives or itching. It could also cause epileptic seizures in susceptible individuals and mental retardation in babies with a genetic tendency toward a disease called phenylketonuria (PKU). In addition, some research indicates that artificial sweeteners may stimulate the appetite, especially for carbohydrates, encouraging overeating. Many doctors advise that artificial sweeteners should be used with caution by young children and pregnant and breastfeeding women.

Many packaged and canned foods contain sugar. Read labels and be aware of "hidden" sugars in foods. More than half the sugar we eat comes from processed food.

SALT

Salt affects the water balance in the body's cells, can be detrimental to the circulatory system and may contribute to a potassium deficiency, digestive and nervous disorders, kidney disease, cancer and high blood pressure. For some people it also stimulates the appetite, leading to over-eating.

Processed food contributes 75 to 80 percent of the sodium in the American diet. Avoid sodium-containing substances such as baking powder, baking soda, monosodium glutamate, sodium benzoate, sodium caseinate, sodium citrate, sodium nitrite, sodium phosphate, sodium propionate and sodium saccharin. Rinsing canned vegetables to which salt has been added can get rid of 40 percent of the sodium, and the sodium content of canned tuna can be lowered 75 to 80 percent by washing the tuna for one minute under tap water.

TOXIC ADDITIVES such as MSG, BHA, BHT, sodium nitrate and nitrite, artificial color and flavor, etc. should be avoided. These additives are extremely stressful to the body, contributing to numerous disorders including cancer, schizophrenia and hyperactivity. A difficult child may be a very sick child—a result of eating adulterated food.

Foods that frequently contain toxic additives are the following:

- Bacon, frankfurters, sausage, liverwurst, pork, bologna, salami, tongue, corned beef, pastrami, smoked fish, gefilte fish, packaged seafood, canned ham.
- Canned soups, soup mixes, canned vegetables, canned sauces, canned tomato paste, bouillon cubes.
- Bottled salad dressings, vegetable shortenings, jams, jellies, mayonnaise, ketchup, meat tenderizers.
- Processed cheeses, frozen pizzas, cheese spreads, butter, margarine.
- Dry roasted nuts, red pistachio nuts.
- Baby formulas.
- Packaged cakes and cake mixes, packaged cookies, crackers, pies, doughnuts, pretzels, pastry icings and fillings, jello, puddings, gelatin, frozen desserts, ice cream, ice milk, whipped toppings, sugar substitutes, chewing gum.
- Colas, soft drinks, chocolate milk, evaporated milk, punches, powders, beer, cocoa, instant teas.

Many of the above listed foods can be purchased in the health food store without toxic additives. However, be sure to read labels even in the health food store, and work toward preparing foods as fresh and as home made as possible.

PROCESSED AND REFINED FLOURS, GRAINS, CEREALS AND PASTA, such as white flour, white rice, etc. These foods are mostly starch, with almost all essential nutrients (vitamins E, B, and other vitamins and minerals, protein, and fiber) removed. They require work and energy to metabolize while giving you no nutrients in return, and they fill you up so that you have no room for the foods that do support you.

"Enriched" grains contain only a few synthetic vitamins, replacing about 25 nutrients removed in processing. Refined products often contain sugar, salt, stabilizers, bleach and other potentially toxic additives.

Use of these foods increases susceptibility to disease. They contribute to obesity, disorders of digestion, metabolism and elimination, to vitamin and mineral deficiency diseases, nervous and other disorders. Evidence shows that lack of fiber in the diet may be a major contributory factor in the rise of colon and other forms of cancer, in hemorrhoids, varicose veins, appendicitis, heart disease, diabetes, and other chronic disorders.

MEATS INJECTED WITH HORMONES, ANTIBIOTICS, AND OTHER CHEMICALS, AND RAISED ON CHEMICAL FEED. Hormones in the meats may contribute to hormonal imbalances in humans, to sterility and cancer. Our excessive consumption of antibiotics, including in our meats, has given rise to a strain of antibiotic resistant bacteria. This may seriously undermine the effectiveness of antibiotics in medicine.

It is not necessary to avoid meat altogether. However, there are four things to consider if you have made the decision to include meat in your diet:

(1) The level of adulteration. Try to avoid meat from animals that are injected with hormones and antibiotics, and are fed chemical

feed. Keep in mind that it is in the liver, skin and fatty portions of the meat that the toxins are particularly concentrated. Also avoid luncheon meats and bacon packaged with nitrates, possible carcinogens.

Whenever possible, get organic meat; that is, meat from animals that have not been injected, and have been raised free-range on their natural feed. Sometimes health food stores and fine meat markets carry organic meat and liver, and hot dogs and bacon without nitrates. Occasionally kosher meat is organic, and lamb is usually not injected.

(2) The level of "natural" contamination. Pork often contains parasites which are extremely resistant to high heat and prolonged cooking. Sometimes raw fish contains parasites, and shellfish can be contaminated. Choose the freshest possible fish from a reputable store or restaurant.

(3) The fat in meat may contribute to heart disease and certain types of cancer. Choose lean meat such as white meat poultry or, if you eat red meat, choose select grade top round, preferably organic. Avoid fatty luncheon meats such as bologna and salami, also high in sodium. Cut off all fatty portions of the meat, and remove the skin of poultry.

(4) The method of cooking. Avoid fried and smoked meats. High heats cause cancer-causing substances in these fats. Choose cooking techniques such as roasting, broiling or grilling. Cook meat on a rack so fat drips away during cooking.

All of these "avoids" concerning meat may sound overwhelming. Again, work with the good, better, best guide. Get the best meat, fish or chicken available. Then enjoy it. If you are primarily eating the high fiber, high nutrient foods listed in Chapter 1, your body should be able to balance out the effects of toxins and fat in the meat.

HIGH HEATED, RANCID, HYDROGENATED AND PROCESSED OILS. Oils heated to high temperatures, particularly beyond 250°, become difficult to digest, irritate the gastrointestinal lining, contribute to heart disease, and are converted to toxic, cancer-causing substances.

When foods are cooked in high-heated oils, such as in high heat frying, barbecuing and smoking, cancer-causing substances are formed in the foods, and polyunsaturated oils are converted to toxins which prevent the utilization of other dietary oils. In cooking with oils, cook with low heat. Use olive oil, canola oil or butter, which are least affected by high heat.

Heating oils also results in a loss of lecithin and many minerals and vitamins, including vitamin E which, in addition to being a vitamin we need for good health, prevents the oil from becoming rancid.

Oils and oil-based foods, such as nuts and seeds, nut butters and wheat germ become rancid at room temperature. Always keep them in the refrigerator or freezer.

Most commercially processed oils are subjected to high heats, bleaching and deodorizing, and contain toxic or questionable chemicals, such as BHA and BHT.

When oils are hydrogenated, or artificially hardened, to produce margarine or shortenings, many vitamins, minerals and essential fatty acids are lost. In addition, the structure of the fat molecule is altered in such a way that it becomes difficult to utilize. Recent evidence suggests that hydrogenated fats may contribute to heart disease.

In summary, when using oils, use oils which have been processed and heated as little as possible. These are the "cold-pressed oils." Remember to cook on low heats.

OILS WHICH ARE DIFFICULT TO DIGEST, such as coconut, palm, cottonseed, safflower, peanut, corn. These oils put tremendous strain on the liver. Soy oil, though one of the better oils nutritionally, is a common allergen and can contribute to congestion, so use it in moderation.

OVERCONSUMPTION OF ALCOHOL encourages birth defects, complications of pregnancy and blood sugar problems. It can destroy brain cells, harm blood vessels, the heart, liver, pancreas, nerves and other organs. It is associated with traffic accidents, domestic violence, depression and child abuse. It depletes the body of nutrients since it draws on our reserves to digest and detoxify, depresses the appetite and interferes with digestion and assimilation.

As a "transition" alcohol, some people more easily tolerate pure vodka with tomato juice and a dash of cayenne pepper. Use less vodka each time, and more tomato juice and cayenne. Cayenne contains calcium, vitamin C and niacin to give you extra support in overcoming the effects of the alcohol.

Eating food, especially protein and raw vegetables, while drinking alcohol also helps reduce the negative effects of the alcohol.

PASTEURIZED, HOMOGENIZED MILK AND ITS PRODUCTS, especially cow's milk, are common allergens, encouraging gastrointestinal disorders, asthma, hay fever, arthritis and other chronic disease, as well as hyperactivity and other behavioral problems. For many people, they are extremely mucus-forming, and are generally congesting.

Heating proteins, such as in pasteurizing milk, decreases digestibility. Some research suggests that homogenized milk may contribute to heart disease.

Commercial milk often contains hormones, antibiotics, radioactive isotopes, pesticides and other pollutants.

See "Foods to Enjoy—Dairy," p. 36, for dairy products that are less stressful.

CAFFEINE- AND TANNIN-CONTAINING BEVERAGES SUCH AS COFFEE, BLACK TEAS AND COLAS. Caffeine is overstimulating to the heart and can aggravate stomach ulcers, nervousness, headaches, and skin, intestinal and other disorders. It also interferes with the use of iron and certain vitamins, and creates vitamin B deficiencies, contributing to stress.

Tannin can damage the liver and mucous membrane of the mouth and digestive tract, interfering with digestion and elimination.

CHOCOLATE is high in fat, calories and sugar, since its natural bitter taste requires excessive sweetening. It contains theobromine and caffeine, which are excessively stimulating to the heart, and oxalic acid which inhibits the metabolism of calcium.

Chocolate is usually an allergen, and may contribute to skin problems, constipation, breathing and digestive difficulties, cystic breast disease, herpes, depressive mood swings and other disorders.

ALLERGENS are foods which can in certain cases trigger allergy symptoms, such as headaches, insomnia, abdominal distress, poor concentration and coordination, anxiety, dizziness, fatigue, asthma, hyperactivity, mood swings with no apparent cause, sudden anger, runny nose, dark circles under the eyes, and an excessive craving for the allergen.

It is as if one is "addicted" to the allergen. Eating it makes one temporarily feel better, since it postpones the withdrawal symptoms, but ultimately perpetuates the addiction syndrome, contributing to further weakness.

The most common food allergens are sugar, artificial food colors, cow's milk, wheat, corn, rye, barley, oats, chocolate, eggs, coffee, cola, peanuts, walnuts, pecans, citrus, beef, pork, bananas, white potatoes, tomatoes, cinnamon, fish, shrimp, onion, garlic, yeast, snap beans and dried peas.

To avoid eating a food allergen is helpful, but it is more important to find out why the body is rejecting the food. Allergic reactions can be caused by lack of digestive enzymes, malnourishment, weak adrenal and digestive function, and overall toxicity. A latent food allergy can manifest from eating too much of one food too often. This is one reason it is so important to vary your foods.

If you suspect a food allergy, avoid the food for five to seven days, then eat it first thing in the morning and see how you respond. There are various other tests, including blood tests, and taking your pulse after eating, which can help you identify the allergens. Consult your nutrition consultant or physician.

13

Low Stress Change

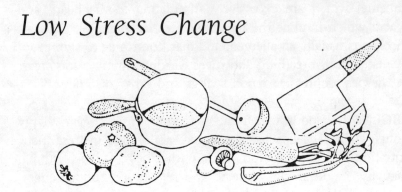

Although there are generally foods which support good health and foods which encourage ill health, diets vary with each person and with different points in each person's life. There is no one target diet appropriate for everyone at all times. We are always more or less in a state of transition.

On the next page is a Transition Chart which is a simple but helpful guide in grasping an over-all picture of which foods are never supportive at any time; which foods are sometimes necessary; and which foods are supportive at any point. (Naturally, there are always exceptions, such as with food sensitivities.)

Column 1 lists "Foods to Avoid," which are stressful to everyone and should be given up as soon as possible.

The foods in column 2, "Acceptable Foods," may be an important part of your health regime, or may be stressful, depending on your particular reaction. Some of these foods may be part of your menus temporarily, and some may be a permanent part of your diet.

The "Vital Foods" in column 3 generally support health and vitality.

Most people find the best diet for them combines foods in columns 2 and 3. They continuously add and subtract foods from column 2 as their needs change, while including most foods from column 3.

Following is a visual representation of the usual progression of a transition:

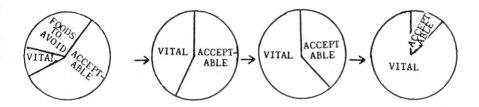

The circle represents your total diet at one time. You should eliminate the "Foods to Avoid" as soon as possible, then gradually cut down on the "Acceptable" foods, but not eliminate them altogether. Again, certain "Acceptable" foods may be as supportive for you as the "Vital" foods. Eating only "Vital" foods should not necessarily be a goal. The ratio of "Acceptable" foods to "Vital" foods is an individual decision. However, your diet should primarily consist of "Vital" foods.

If the "Foods to Avoid" make up a major part of your diet, and you are in a state of shock at the prospect of eliminating them immediately, don't be discouraged. "Immediately" really means as soon as possible, but it may take you a while to eliminate them altogether. There will probably be times when it is relatively easy for you to avoid them. Then, many times you will slip because of the social situation you are in, or because of old habits and cravings. Keep working at it. Eventually you will lose your taste for them. (Honest! Even I did.) At that point you simply won't want or need to eat them.

Remember that there are many delicious foods which will more than replace these non-foods, and which will make your transition easier and more enjoyable than you can imagine. It is simply a matter of education, experimentation and discovery.

Your increased health and vitality will also give you the encouragement to take the next steps.

TRANSITION CHART

FOODS TO AVOID	FOODS TO ENJOY	
Eliminate Immediately	**Acceptable Foods** *Experiment with These*	**Vital Foods** *Primarily Use These*
PROTEINS		
Meats with additives, such as luncheon meat packed with nitrites (bologna, salami, etc) Processed cheese Battery eggs Battery chicken *Raised in small coops, injected with antibiotics, etc.* Meat with hormones, etc. Pork; veal Pasteurized, homogenized cow's milk Yogurt with sugar, and toxic additives	Meat without additives, hormones, antibiotics, etc., raised free-range on organic feed Deep ocean or pure-lake fish Certified raw milk Raw cheese Yogurt without toxic additives Raw soured milk Cultured buttermilk Cottage cheese without toxic additives Dry milk powder without toxic additives	Sprouts Fresh, raw nuts and seeds: flax, chia, pumpkin, sunflower, sesame, almond, pecan, brazil, walnut, filbert, etc. Nut butters Nut milks Organic eggs Beans: lentils, soy beans, split peas, black beans, etc. Tofu, tempeh
CARBOHYDRATES		
Sugar: white, brown, turbinado, sucrose, glucose, corn syrup, fructose, etc. Chocolate Processed carbohydrates such as white flour and white flour products White rice Anything packaged or canned with sugar, salt or toxic additives Processed pasta Ice cream with sugar and toxic additives	Raw honey; unsulphured molasses; barley malt; pure maple syrup Carob Whole grain Bread Whole grain Pasta Pure ice cream made without toxic additives or sugar	Vegetables: squash, carrots, celery, tomatoes, beets, cabbage, broccoli, cauliflower, leeks, turnips, radish, lettuce, etc. Fruit: apple, grapes, bananas, papayas, pineapple, peach, melon, etc. Sea vegetables Whole grains: brown rice, millet, rye, barley, etc.

Foods to Avoid	Foods to Enjoy	
Eliminate Immediately	**Acceptable Foods** *Experiment with These*	**Vital Foods** *Primarily Use These*
LIPIDS		
Oils that are rancid or overheated Rancid animal fats, such as lard, bacon drippings, etc. Anything deep-fat fried Artificially hardened fats, such as margarine and shortenings	Oils which are not rancid or overheated Unsalted butter	Raw, cold-pressed oils: olive, sunflower, sesame, flax, almond, walnut, avocado, soy, canola Raw, unsalted butter Avocado Fresh, raw nuts and seeds
OTHER		
Coffee, tannic-acid teas; excess alcohol Common table salt Any commercial condiments with sugar, salt or toxic additives Commercial soft drinks made with toxic additives and sugar	Pure grain coffee substitutes Not more than 1 glass a day of non-chemicalized wine or beer Aluminum-free baking powder Soft drinks made without chemicals, sugar or toxic additives Soy sauce without toxic additives Potassium balanced salt; sea salt Vegetable salt and kelp	Herb teas and seasonings Organic apple cider vinegar Home-made condiments without salt or sugar Freshly juiced vegetables and fruits Fresh fruit ice cream Spring water

14

Practical Tips For A Smooth Transition: Converting and Supplementing Recipes

Psychologically as well as physically it is easier to adapt to a new diet if you begin with recipes to which you are accustomed, but with healthful changes.

You can convert old recipes, substituting healthful ingredients for stressful ones, such as whole wheat flour for white flour, and you can supplement old recipes with ingredients which add flavor and a nutritional boost.

An added bonus for converting and supplementing recipes: You will be happily surprised at how much more delicious your recipes will be!

CONVERT YOUR RECIPES

In converting recipes, you can totally replace processed ingredients (such as sugar, white flour, white rice, white pasta) with natural sweeteners and whole grain ingredients, following the simple guide-lines on the next few pages.

You can also add the whole grain ingredients gradually, using a mixture of processed and whole grain until you and your family are accustomed to the new color and taste. For example, mix brown and white rice to-gether, whole wheat and white flour, whole grain and white pasta.

Following are some guidelines for converting your recipes.

You will note that I have included conversion tips for whole wheat flour to other flours, and for eggs to other ingredients. Although whole wheat and eggs are normally good foods, many people are allergic to wheat and eggs, as well as dairy, and need substitutes.

HOW TO CHANGE YOUR RECIPES

Sugar to Honey

In beverages: to taste

In baking:

Use ½ to ¾ cup honey for 1 cup sugar, depending on how sweet you want it (usually ½).

Reduce the amount of liquid in the recipe ¼ cup for each cup of honey used. For example, if ½ cup of honey is used, reduce the liquid by 2 tablespoons.

In cakes which call for no liquid, where crispness is important, add 4 tablespoons additional flour for every 1 cup honey.

Lower the oven temperature by about 25° since honey browns more quickly than sugar.

To make it easier to measure the honey without having it stick to the measuring cup, lightly oil the cup first. Or, if the recipe calls for oil, measure the oil first.

If you wish to liquefy honey for easier measuring and blending, gently warm it.

Sugar to Molasses

In beverages: to taste

In baking:
   Usually, molasses, rather than honey, is used in place of brown sugar.
   Use ½ to ¾ c. molasses in place of brown sugar.
   Reduce the amount of liquid in the recipe by ¼ cup for each cup of molasses.

Note: When a recipe calls for 1 cup white sugar and 1 cup brown sugar, use ¾ cup honey and ¼ cup molasses.

Salt to Soy Sauce, such as Tamari, or to Powdered Seaweed, such as Kelp or Dulse Powder, or to Salt-Free Vegetable "Salt"

To taste. Begin with small amounts. Keep in mind that kelp and soy sauce will turn the food a darker color, and that kelp has a "seaweed" taste. If you are allergic to wheat, make sure your soy sauce is wheat-free.
   As a very first step, you may want to use sea salt in place of common table salt. Use it to taste. Sea salt has no chemicals added to it to make it flow freely, and has been dried naturally in the sun.

Chocolate to Carob

In recipes that call for solid chocolate, use 3 tablespoons carob powder plus 2 tablespoons water or nut milk to one square of chocolate. (One square is usually equal to one ounce.)
   Be sure to use carob powder that has no added sugar. There is also roasted and unroasted carob powder. Most people prefer the roasted.
   Carob dissolves better in oil than in water.
   To help get rid of the raw taste of carob, mix it with *hot* liquid.
   Ground filbert nuts, vanilla extract and a little molasses help to give carob more of a "chocolate" taste. However, carob can be delicious in its own right. Don't expect it to taste just like chocolate, and you won't be disappointed.

White Flour to Whole Wheat Flour

In general, remove 2 tablespoons of whole wheat flour for every 1 cup of white flour, particularly with *sifted* white flour.

For example, 2 cups *sifted* white flour equals 1¾ cups *sifted* whole wheat flour. And, 2 cups *unsifted* white flour equals 2 cups *sifted* whole wheat flour.

If you are using coarse ground wheat, remove 2 tablespoons whole wheat flour for every one cup of white flour. Omit sifting. Just stir lightly.

Whole wheat pastry flour is lighter, and better suited for cakes and cookies than whole wheat flour. Use the same proportions as for whole wheat.

Whole Wheat Flour to Other Flours

Although whole wheat is a nutritious grain, many people have wheat allergies.

For 1 cup of wheat flour use any of the following:

1¼ c. rye flour
½ c. rye flour + ½ c. potato flour
⅔ c. rye flour + ⅓ c. cooked potato
1 c. millet flour
½ c. millet flour and ½ c. cooked potato (either white or sweet, depending on the taste you want)
¼ c. ground nuts and/or seeds + ¾ c. cooked potato
¾ c. cooked potato + 2 Tbl. soy flour
1 c. corn flour
⅞ c. rice flour
½ c. rice flour + ½ c. oat flour
¼ c. amaranth flour + ¾ c. brown rice or oat flour

Notes on Converting Whole Wheat to Other Flours:

Millet flour has a "bite" to it so it is best in recipes with an ingredient which can overpower it such as in a spice cake or a banana bread.

If you use potato flour or cooked potato, you may need to increase the liquid amount. If you use cooked potato, measure by quickly grinding it in the blender. Blend the cooked potato with the liquid and spices, then add to the dry ingredients. Millet flour or ground nuts work well with cooked potato.

Soy flour is difficult to digest and has a strong, slightly unpleasant taste, so it is best not to use more than 2 tablespoons to a cup, or ⅛ of your total flour volume.

Since soy is high in protein and fat, it causes heavy browning of the crust. Therefore, if you use a large amount of soy flour, reduce the oven temperature by 25°.

Since soy flour is high in fat, it should be mixed with the wet ingredients rather than the dry.

Soy flour acts as a preservative. Breads made with it stay fresh longer.

A small amount of soy flour in your breads will make them a more complete protein.

Rice flour is quite heavy, so it is best mixed with another, lighter flour. In addition, beating the egg whites till they form soft peaks, and folding them into the batter, will make the cake, bread, muffins, etc. lighter in texture.

White Rice to Brown Rice

Use the same amounts, but plan on more cooking time, depending on the method used.

Milk to "Nut Milk"

Nut Milk is a milky looking liquid made by blending ground nuts and/or seeds, or nut butter, with water. Nut milk can be used in place of milk in any recipe and will add the taste of the nut or seed.

Almond milk, which has a delicious, mild flavor, is particularly good in place of milk.

Use the same amounts of nut milk as you would cow's milk.

Raw goat's milk is often well tolerated in place of cow's milk.

However, it is difficult to find and, although some goat's milk is delicious, especially when fresh, the taste is often disliked.

Eggs to other ingredients

For one egg use any of the following:

    1 teaspoon arrowroot flour
    1 teaspoon yam flour
    1 teaspoon sweet rice flour

Or for baking, use 1 tablespoon lecithin for 1 egg. Blend it fast with an oil included in the recipe. Then, if the recipe calls for a sweetener, blend with that.

Or to cold water add 1 cup ground flaxseed. Bring to a boil, stirring constantly. Boil for 3 minutes. Let cool, then place in the refrigerator in a closed jar. Whenever your recipe calls for 1 beaten egg, substitute 1 tablespoon of the above mixture.

Or dissolve 1 package unflavored gelatin in hot water. Two to three tablespoons will work well in cheesecakes and pies.

Or soak ½ pound apricots in 2 cups water overnight. The next morning, blend them. Add water, if needed. Strain and store in the refrigerator. Every time your recipe calls for beaten eggs, take a generous tablespoon of apricot purée and blend with your recipe.

Animal Fats, Lard, Shortening to Butter

Use 1 cup butter in place of any of the following:

    2 cups commercial shortening
    1 cup margarine
    ⁴/₅ cup bacon fat (clarified)
    ³/₄ cup chicken fat
    ⁷/₈ cup cottonseed, corn, nut oil
    ⁷/₈ cup lard
    ⁴/₅ to ⁷/₈ cup drippings

Note that sesame butter or tahini can be used as a shortening for bread or cookies in place of butter or other fat.

ENRICHING YOUR RECIPES

Another tip for making your transition smooth and your recipes more delicious and power-packed, is to supplement them with ingredients which add nourishment.

SUPPLEMENTS TO ENRICH YOUR MEALS

SUPPLEMENT	SPECIAL NUTRIENT	ADD IT TO
Bran (wheat or rice)	Fiber	Breads, cakes, cookies, cereals, beverages and blender drinks, loaves, casseroles, etc.
Cayenne pepper	Vitamin C; calcium	Add after cooking to vegetable juice, soups, steamed vegetables, grains, sauces, dressings, etc.
Kelp or dulse powder	Iodine and other minerals	Use whenever you would use salt, but would not mind a light seaweed taste.
Molasses (unsulfured)	Potassium, iron, trace minerals	Add to water as a beverage; in blender drinks, cereals, cookies, etc. (Don't overdo.)
Nutritional yeast	Vitamin B complex	Beverages, blender drinks, bread, cookies, soups, loaves and casseroles, burgers, etc.
Nuts & seeds: whole, ground, or as milks	Protein and many vitamins and minerals	Casseroles, loaves, burgers, cereals, breads, beverages and blender drinks, sauces, dressings, snacks, on salads and desserts.
Parsley	Vitamin A & C; iron and other minerals	Juices, soups, dressings, sauces, salads, vegetables, loaves, burgers, grains, beans, meats, etc.
Rice polishings	Silicon and vitamin B complex	Beverages, blender drinks, bread, cookies, soups, loaves, burgers, casseroles, sauces, etc.

Supplement	Special Nutrient	Add It To
Soy powder	Protein; B vitamins	Beverages and blender drinks, soups, casseroles, loaves, bread, cookies, etc. (Don't overdo. It's hard to digest.)
Sprouts	Enzymes, protein, vitamins A, C and many other vitamins, minerals and fiber	Salads, sandwiches, sauces, dressings, soups, omelettes, loaves, etc. Add last to hot things. Don't cook, if possible, as cooking kills many of the nutrients.
Wheat germ (vacuum packed)	B vitamins, vitamin E, protein, potassium and phosphorus	Beverages and blender drinks, breads, cookies, cakes, cereals, loaves and casseroles, burgers, on salads or desserts.

15

Equipment & Utensils

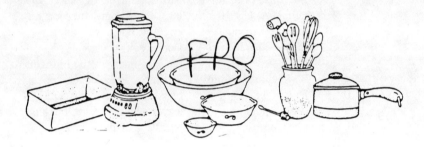

The equipment and utensils used in the preparation of foods can save time, and can help you prepare food that is packed with nutrition.

The following pages contain pictures, and a listing of the most basic equipment and utensils. Some of them can be used in the following ways:

Flame tamer: Extremely helpful for low-heat cooking. It is simply a wire frame or fire-proof pad designed to buffer the heat between the stove top and the pot. If you cannot locate one in a store, make your own with a wire or wire hanger.

Blender: Wonderful for making smoothies, green drinks, blended salads, nut milks, grain water, creamy cereals, sauces, dips, dressings, fruit ice creams, soups, etc. Most people find that a simple blender with four speeds is sufficient.

Juicer: Extracts juice from fruits or vegetables. There are various types of juicers. The "press type" is preferable for best preserving food nutrients, although other kinds may be simpler to use. Some types also double for mashing frozen fruits into ice creams, or sprouted grains into breads.

Grater: To grate raw vegetables such as carrots, beets, sweet potatoes for making salads, loaves, etc.

Nut-seed grinder: To grind nuts and seeds for nut milks, nut/seed loaves or patties, or to add to breads, salads, cereals, etc. It also grinds grains or beans as flour for cereals and breads.

Steamer: For steaming vegetables, heating cooked grains or noodles, etc.

Garlic press: For mincing garlic.

Timer: Helps prevent over-cooked food.

Vegetable brush: Handy for scrubbing skins of vegetables that should be eaten with skins (when not heavily sprayed with pesticides) such as carrots, potatoes, Jerusalem artichokes (sunchokes).

Please Note:

Do not cook with aluminum or copper cookware as there is some evidence that they leach toxic levels of metal into the food and pull "life energy" from the food. High levels of aluminum have been shown to impair the nervous system, contributing to liver and kidney failure.

Stainless steel, pyrex, iron, black steel or enamel is best.

If you use black steel, turn the oven down 10° since it absorbs and holds heat more than other cookware.

If you use enamel, be sure it is not chipped.

EQUIPMENT & UTENSILS

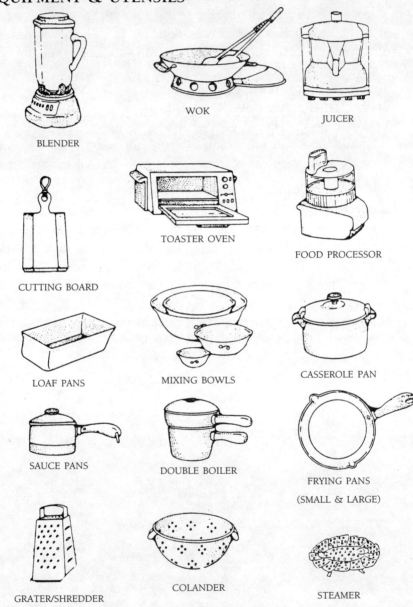

BLENDER

WOK

JUICER

CUTTING BOARD

TOASTER OVEN

FOOD PROCESSOR

LOAF PANS

MIXING BOWLS

CASSEROLE PAN

SAUCE PANS

DOUBLE BOILER

FRYING PANS
(SMALL & LARGE)

GRATER/SHREDDER

COLANDER

STEAMER

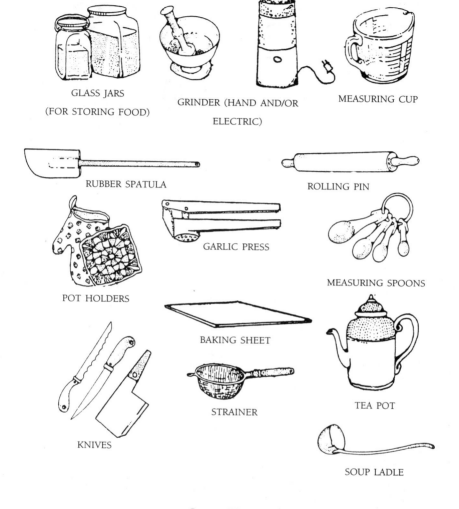

GLASS JARS
(FOR STORING FOOD)

GRINDER (HAND AND/OR ELECTRIC)

MEASURING CUP

RUBBER SPATULA

ROLLING PIN

GARLIC PRESS

POT HOLDERS

MEASURING SPOONS

BAKING SHEET

KNIVES

STRAINER

TEA POT

SOUP LADLE

OTHER UTENSILS

sprouting equipment (glass jar, cheese cloth, rubber band)

spoons (stainless & wooden)

asbestos pad or flame tamer

timer
wire whisk
spatula
tea kettle
crock pot

water filter
kitchen shears
vegetable brush
wooden salad bowl

16

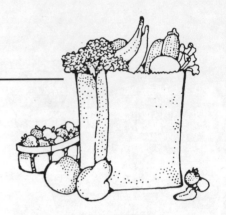

Shopping Hints

Easy shopping and a knowledge of which staples to have on hand adds to stress-free food preparation. Here are some hints:

(1) Buy grain, flour, dried beans, nuts, and seeds in bulk. Put grains, flour, nuts and seeds in covered glass or porcelain jars in the refrigerator to keep them fresh. Nuts and seeds keep even better in the freezer.

(2) When you buy ingredients for a meal, you may want to buy extra, to prepare something for the next day.

(3) Try to buy perishable foods as close to a meal as possible.

(4) Note staples necessary for the meal that may be low.

(5) Note foods already on hand.

STAPLES

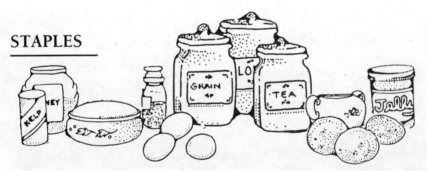

These are foods which keep well, which you can have on hand all the time. Be sure they are as unadulterated as possible.

Staples can be divided into three categories:

A. Those which store well over a long period of time. These can be purchased once a month, or even less frequently.

B. Those which keep fairly well. These can be purchased once a week.

C. The more perishable foods, such as certain fruits and vegetables, which may need to be purchased every couple of days. These are not included on this list.

GROUP A—STAPLES TO PURCHASE ONCE A MONTH, OR LESS

Beverages: grain coffee substitutes, herb teas, pure bottled juices, spring or distilled water.

Cereals*: home-made granola or good quality store bought.

Seasonings: herbs and spices; herb and vegetable salt substitutes; apple cider vinegar*; soy sauce; kelp powder; onions, garlic.

Crackers: rice, rye and/or wheat.

Dried beans: aduki, garbanzo, kidney, lentil, split pea, mung, etc.

Dried fruit: (unsulfured) raisins, dates, figs, etc.

Extracts: pure vanilla, orange, almond.

Flour*: whole grain rye, wheat, pastry wheat, millet, etc.

Grains*: brown rice, millet, whole wheat and/or rye berries, barley, corn meal, rolled oats, rye flakes, bulgur (cracked wheat), buckwheat.

Miscellaneous*: sugar-free jams, mayonnaise, ketchup, popcorn, miso, agar agar, kuzu. (Refrigerate all except kuzu and agar agar.)

Pasta: whole wheat, buckwheat, Jerusalem artichoke, quinoa, amaranth, and other wheat-free pasta.

Nutritional supplements:* nutritional yeast, bran, vacuum packed wheat germ, rice polishings, etc.

Nuts & seeds:* almonds, sunflower, chia, flax, sesame, pumpkin, alfalfa (to sprout), etc.

Oils:* cold pressed olive, sunflower, sesame, walnut, soy, canola

*Refrigerate

Soups: vegetable powders and bouillon cubes.

Sweeteners: honey, maple syrup, molasses, barley malt, rice bran syrup, unsweetened carob powder.

Seaweed: dulse, wakame, nori, etc.

GROUP B—STAPLES TO PURCHASE ONCE A WEEK

*Bread:** whole grain, home-made or good store-bought.

*Butter:** unsalted dairy butter and seed butters, such as tahini or almond butter.

*Eggs:** organic.

*Freezer items:** chicken, fish, nut/seed burgers.

*Vegetables:** those that keep well: potatoes, carrots, radish, parsnips, turnips, sunchokes (Jerusalem artichokes), squash.

*Fruits:** those that keep well: apples, pears and other hard fruits.

*Refrigerate.

As you can see, this is quite an extensive list, even though it does not include the third category of staples—the more perishable foods (leafy greens and the more delicate fruits and vegetables)! With such a variety of foods from this staples list—whole grains, pasta, beans, nuts and seeds, frozen chicken and fish, certain vegetables and fruits, condiments and flavorings—many different delicious meals can be created with very little daily shopping. This saves time and food waste and stimulates your own creative instincts.

17

Planning Your Meals

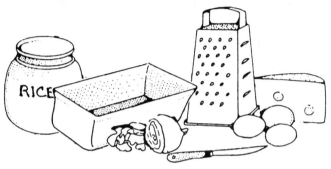

In planning your meals there are a few basic considerations to keep in mind:

- The availability of foods
- The cost of food
- Spoilage
- Preparation time
- For whom are you cooking?
- The weather
- Calories
- The over-all plan of the meal, which should include good taste, moderation, simplicity, balance, variety and vitality.
- The basic food elements included in a daily menu—protein, vitamins, minerals, oils, fiber, chlorophyll.
- Proportions of food categories: How many vegetables, fruits, grains, proteins to include in a day.
- Combining vegetarian proteins to increase net protein utilization. See Chapter 18.
- How to combine and consume foods for better digestion and assimilation. See Chapter 19.

Planning your meals well simply means using your common sense. Learn to develop your ability to listen to the magical voice inside you.

In planning your meals, it is important to consider the availability of the foods, the cost and spoilage factors, preparation time, and cooking for others. In addition, the following factors should be considered:

WEATHER

Your body will adapt more easily to a new diet if you choose lighter foods (such as more fruits and vegetables) in summer, and heavier foods (such as whole grains and beans) in winter. If possible, use foods that are grown in your region. Those foods have within them all that is needed to survive in that climate, and that factor is transferred to you.

CALORIES

Foods are likely to be high in calories if they are:

- Greasy or oily: butter, fried foods (such as potato chips or french fries); foods cooked in large amounts of fat;
- Smooth and thick: rich sauces, cream cheese, mayonnaise, tartar sauce, sour cream, avocado, nut butters (peanut butter, tahini, almond butter), cream;
- Sweet and gooey: candy, regular soft drinks, rich baked goods, ice cream;
- Alcoholic

A food is less likely to be high in calories if it is:

• Thin and watery, like tomato juice;
• An unadorned vegetable or fruit

Foods highest in calories are those containing fat, since fat has more than twice as many calories ounce for ounce as protein or carbohydrates (grains, beans, fruits and vegetables.) In addition, in the process of digesting, metabolizing and storing foods, the body burns more calories processing carbohydrates such as grains and beans than it does fat. So, for a given number of calories, you'll gain more weight from fat.

High-fat foods include butter, mayonnaise and oil, meat, nuts and seeds, fried food, cheese, ice cream, avocado and foods with "hidden" fats such as cakes, muffins, cookies, and granola.

Low-fat foods include fruits, vegetables, whole grains and beans.

When considering the caloric value of foods, keep in mind how it affects the appetite and over-all health. Certain foods that are high in calories may be beneficial for our health. For example, certain fats such as olive oil, avocados, almonds, walnuts and fatty fish (salmon, sardines, mackerel) may help prevent heart disease, diabetes, arthritis and skin problems, while other fats, such as butter, cheese and meat may encourage heart disease and certain types of cancer.

Although some people are concerned about the calories in whole grains, beans and potatoes, these foods are very low in fat. They are also high in fiber and essential nutrients, helping satisfy the appetite, which reduces over-eating. These nutrient-dense foods supply the body with protein, vitamins and minerals that are more than worth the caloric "cost." Foods high in sugar and salt, on the other hand, stimulate the appetite, causing one to over-eat.

As you cut out "junk" food and begin to eat more and more "real" food, your body will slim down naturally.

A MEAL PLAN

When we are first making a conscious effort to have a diet plan, it helps to be aware of how we have been eating up to now. To assist you in becoming aware of your eating habits, fill out a chart for a week, with a format something like the one below:

DAILY DIET REPORT							
	1ST DAY	2ND DAY	3RD DAY	4TH DAY	5TH DAY	6TH DAY	7TH DAY
MORNING MEAL							
NOON MEAL							
EVENING MEAL							
SNACKS							
COMMENTS							

Commenting on each day's food intake can help expand your awareness of the effects of your diet on your over-all health. This column can include reactions you may have after a meal—physical symptoms, including sleepiness, or emotional swings. You may want to note circumstances surrounding the meal, including eating under stress, fighting at a meal, etc. Working with this column can help you discover food allergies, and help you better understand food cravings and your relationship with your food.

When you plan your meal, key points to keep in mind are good taste, moderation, balance, simplicity, variety and vitality.

GOOD TASTE

Don't just eat food because it's healthy. Make it delicious, and appetizing.

MODERATION

When giving up meat, milk, salt and sugar, don't overdo on nuts, cheese, tofu, soy sauce, honey, molasses, yogurt and whole wheat bread. Be moderate. Overconsumption of these foods (i.e., every day or twice a day) can encourage mucous build up, digestive stress, allergies or other stress reactions.

BALANCE

Balance your meals by varying the color, texture, flavor and shape of individual foods. This is Mother Nature's way of helping you get a good range and balance of food value, as well as making it more appealing to the eye and taste buds.

SIMPLICITY

Use the "KISS" Rule: Keep It Simple, Sweetheart.

Preparing two to three items per meal will be easiest on your digestion, time and energy.

Although it is always best to prepare foods fresh, sometimes making extra for the next day will cut down on stress, and help prevent one from eating junk food.

VARIETY

Most deficiency diseases result from not getting enough variety in the diet, rather than a lack of one specific nutrient.

Vary your vegetables, fruits, grains, beans, nuts and seeds and oils from day to day. This makes your meals more interesting, gives you a greater balance of nutrients, and helps prevent food allergies (sometimes aggravated from eating a food too much and too often).

Sometimes we are not aware of how often we repeat the same foods over and over. This is usually because we don't have the time or energy to experiment with something different. Filling out the diet plan for one week helps with this awareness.

Learning a few basic techniques, such as those outlined in Chapter 20, can free you from the stress of thinking about recipes, yet leave room for variety.

VITALITY

Choose foods that give you vitality—the "Foods to Enjoy" listed in Chapter 11.

FOOD ELEMENTS FOR A DAILY MENU

In planning your meal, be sure it provides you with the following elements:

ELEMENT	FOOD SOURCE
enzymes	raw vegetables and fruits, sprouts
fiber	whole grains, dried beans and peas, fruits and vegetables, nuts and seeds, sprouts
chlorophyll	dark green vegetables such as broccoli, kale, romaine lettuce, spinach, Swiss chard, watercress, peas, alfalfa sprouts, etc.

protein	lamb, chicken, fish, eggs, cheese, yogurt, beans, whole grains, sprouts, nuts and seeds
vitamins	all of the above, plus all cooked or raw vegetables or fruit
minerals	all of the above, plus all cooked or raw vegetables or fruit
quality oils	nuts and seeds, avocados, fish, olive oil, sunflower oil, sesame oil, soy oil, walnut oil, flaxseed oil, canola oil

PROPORTIONS OF FOOD CATEGORIES IN A DAY

To support overall good health, include in a day's meal the following proportions of food types:

5 to 9 servings of vegetables each day

A serving means 1 cup of leafy vegetables; ½ cup of other vegetables (cooked or raw) or ¾ cup of vegetable juice. Try to have at least three different vegetables daily, including a minimum of two green vegetables per day (such as Romaine lettuce, broccoli, peas or kale); two yellow or orange vegetables (such as carrots, winter squash or sweet potato); and one red vegetable (such as beet, tomato or red cabbage). At first glance, this may seem like a lot of vegetables, but consider that in a salad alone you can easily have many varieties. Make a "rainbow salad."

Include a good portion of your vegetables in a raw state, since this will give you more vitamins, enzymes and fiber. If possible, 60 percent raw vegetables is recommended. Introduce them gradually to avoid getting stomach discomfort from too much fiber too soon.

1 to 4 servings of fruit each day

A serving includes 1 medium apple, banana or orange, or ½ cup of chopped cooked or canned fruit or ¾ cup of fruit juice.

Enjoy a variety of fruits, limiting only the citrus (oranges and grapefruit) since they are often too acidic. Opt for the fruit itself rather than the juice. The fruit contains fiber missing in the juice. Fiber helps prevent chronic disease and also slows down the body's absorption of the fruit sugar, putting less stress on our body's sugar-regulating mechanisms.

Note that most people who eat only fruit in the morning get weak and dizzy until they eat something else. Fruit is best eaten as a snack or dessert.

1 to 3 servings of dairy or its equivalent

A serving is 1 or 2 cups of milk or yogurt (preferably non-fat) or a serving of 1½ or 2 ounces of low-fat cheese per day. If you cannot tolerate cow's milk products, there are ample amounts of calcium in dark leafy greens, sesame seeds, sea vegetables, legumes, and sardines or canned salmon (with the bones).

6 to 11 servings of grains each day

This may sound like a lot of grain, but a serving is only ½ cup of cooked cereal, rice, pasta, or grain sprouts, or 1 ounce of ready-to-eat cereal, 1 slice of bread, or 3 to 4 small crackers.

Try to use a variety of whole grains whenever possible to give you that extra fiber and nutritional value.

2 to 3 servings of protein each day

This includes any of the following:

- 2 to 3 ounces of lean meat, poultry or fish

- ½ cup of cooked dried beans, such as lentils, kidney beans, bean sprouts or chick peas
- 1 egg

Note that 1 ounce of nut butter such as peanut or almond butter equals 1 ounce of lean meat in its protein value.

If you are a vegetarian and are choosing beans and nut butters as your sources of protein, you'll need to be sure to include plenty of whole grains as well, to give you adequate amounts of protein. In general, four servings of whole grains plus two servings of beans and a tablespoon of nuts and seeds should provide a vegetarian with adequate protein for a day.

The type and amount of protein, as with the diet in general, depends on each individual—her over-all health status (including any special situation such as pregnancy), age, body size, climate, type and amount of activity and stress level. In general, four to six ounces of meat, poultry or fish in one day would provide adequate protein. More than that may be harmful due to the fat in those foods. The advantage in choosing vegetarian proteins such as beans and grains is that they are low in fat and high in fiber as well as essential nutrients. Consult with your nutrition consultant concerning your protein needs.

18

Protein in a Vegetarian Diet

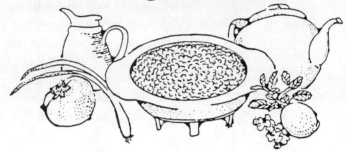

Nuts and seeds, sprouts, whole grains, beans and peas can provide adequate protein, especially when eaten in certain combinations within a period of 12–16 hours. They are also more economical than meat, are high in fiber and low in fat, contain no cholesterol, and are less likely to contain toxic additives.

Don't depend on cheese and tofu for your protein. Over-abundance of these types of high fat protein can be congesting. Tofu has more fat than white meat chicken, although it is a healthy type of fat. Vary your proteins, and learn how to combine them.

Nuts and seeds, beans and grains can be sprouted or eaten in certain combinations to increase the protein utilized from these foods.

Sprouting increases the nutrient value of a nut, seed, legume or grain and also pre-digests the protein so that it is more fully assimilated. All sprouts except buckwheat and sunflower sprouts should be cooked in order to neutralize naturally occurring toxins in the beans and seeds.

Combining nuts and seeds, beans and peas, whole grains and dairy at the same meal or at least within 12–16 hours, can also increase the amount of utilizable protein assimilated from each of the foods.

A simple formula to use is called "Slugem." This formula is a way to remember the letters S-L-G-M, the first letters of the words Seeds, Legumes (beans), Grains and Milk products. Combining foods in the following orders of sequence will give you a more complete protein:

- seeds or nuts with legumes
- legumes with grains
- grains with milk products

Combining seeds and/or nuts with grains increases the net protein utilized, but is not quite as complete as the other combinations.

Following is a list of foods to help you in combining. Note that each category also includes the by-products made from the particular kind of food. For example, included with seeds are seed/nut butters and seed/nut milks.

COMBINING PROTEINS

SEEDS & NUTS +	LEGUMES (BEANS) +	GRAINS +	MILK
sesame seeds	lentils	rice	milk
tahini (sesame	split peas	millet	cheese
butter)	soy beans	barley	yogurt
almonds	mung beans	oats	kefir
almond butter	other beans and	buckwheat	
sunflower seeds	peas	rye	
pumpkin seeds	bean flour, such as	other grains	
flax seeds	soy flour	grain flour	
walnuts	soy products:	noodles, pasta	
pecans	soy sauce	grain milk	
other nuts and seeds	miso	whole grain bread &	
nut milks	tofu	crackers	
	tempeh		

Reading This Chart

Eaten within 16 hours, the following combinations of foods will together make a complete protein:

Seeds & Nuts	+ Legumes	= complete protein
Legumes	+ Grains	= complete protein
Grains	+ Milk products	= complete protein

Nuts and seeds plus grains is a more complete protein than either nuts and seeds alone, or grains alone, but is not as complete a protein as the combinations above.

Notes & Examples:

(1) In general, combine 3 parts grain to 1 part legume.

(2) Adding a small amount of bean flour to grain flour increases the protein used. Even as little as 2 tablespoons of soy flour added to 3 cups of whole wheat or rye flour increases the net protein utilized.

(3) Examples of good combinations are:
   (a) Miso/tahini spread on a rice cracker
   (b) Tofu + noodles with tahini sauce
   (c) Split pea soup and whole grain crackers
   (d) Lentil soup and a rice casserole
   (e) Glass of nut milk and a tofu dip on mixed raw vegetables

19

Combining Foods for Better Digestion

Ideally, we should be able to eat foods in any combination at any time of the day, and digest them well. Many people, however, experience digestive stress in the form of gas, bloating, poor or infrequent bowel movements, overall fatigue, etc. For them, it is of first importance to find out *why* the digestive capacity is weak. Consult with your nutrition consultant or doctor.

Until your digestion is strong again, it is often helpful to avoid eating certain types and combinations of foods which don't digest as easily, and even to be aware of how and when to eat.

TYPES OF FOODS

When first changing your diet, raw foods can sometimes be irritating and you may experience gas. Introduce them gradually or try blending the foods, grating them, or lightly steaming a portion of them . . . especially the harder vegetables. But be sure to have some raw leafy greens each day.

Other types of foods can in and of themselves be gassy, such as cabbage, broccoli, garlic, onions, Brussels sprouts, peppers, and beans. Beans can be blended or cooked in a special way to cut down on the gassy effect. See pp. 242–3.

Nuts and seeds and dried fruit also need to be broken down well, by soaking or blending, and by chewing well.

FOOD COMBINING FOR EASIER DIGESTION

I have found that certain basic combinations eaten at the same meal can cause stress. They are the following:

Often Difficult Combinations:

(1) CERTAIN PROTEIN FOODS + STARCH:

Animal protein + starch (except fish + rice); for example, meat
  plus potatoes, grain or bread
Nuts, seeds, or nut butters + starch; for example, nut butter on bread
Eggs + starch; for example, eggs + bread, or eggs + cereal
Cheese + starch; for example, cheese on bread, or cheese + pasta

(2) CERTAIN PROTEIN FOODS + FRUIT (except tomatoes and the tropical fruits, such as papaya, mango and pineapple):

Meat + fruit (except tomatoes)
Nuts & seeds + fruit
Eggs + fruit
Dairy + fruit; for example, yogurt + fruit, or cheese + fruit

Some people also have difficulty combining fruits with vegetables (except tomatoes, avocados and the tropical fruits).

Easily Digested Combinations:

In general, the best combinations for those with delicate digestion are the following:

Animal protein + vegetables
Starch + vegetables
Fruit is best eaten by itself
Melons are best eaten alone

Sometimes soaked raisins and fresh bananas combine well with starch such as cereals and breads.

Tomatoes and avocados, although fruits, combine well with vegetables and meats.

How long should you wait before you can eat another category of food that does not combine well? It depends on the individual, but basically when you feel hungry again. Usually, you need to wait at least ½ hour after eating fruit before another type of food, and 1 to 1½ hours after protein before eating starch or fruit. This includes dessert, which usually consists of fruit or a starch-containing pastry.

Please note that it is most important to find out *why* the digestive capacity is weak. Avoiding difficult combinations of foods helps give the body a rest, but is not a solution.

TIMING OF FOODS FOR BETTER DIGESTION AND ASSIMILATION

Most people feel better when they eat a power-packed breakfast, a moderate lunch and a light dinner. (Breakfast like a king, lunch like a prince, and dinner like a pauper.)

It is not necessary to have a large breakfast. However, to sustain your energy throughout the day, it helps to have a breakfast that is high in protein, and low in sweets. Sometimes even grains, such as oatmeal for breakfast can be too sweet for some people, leaving them fatigued mid-morning or afternoon. (This could be an "aller-gic" reaction.) Topping your cereals with nut milk, and having a green salad with the cereal may help combat this reaction.

Those with delicate digestion or blood sugar imbalance may find that they have trouble digesting more concentrated proteins, such as beans and meats, after 3 P.M. For them, having that type of protein for lunch rather than dinner helps combat digestive stress and fatigue.

EATING TO AID DIGESTION

Eating your food without stress can be the most important factor in digesting and assimilating all the nutrients possible. Be aware of the following:

(1) Eat only when you are hungry.

(2) Do not feel you must eat when you are sick. It is generally best not to eat, especially if you do not feel like it!

(3) It is best not to eat when you are tired or have negative emotions such as anger, guilt, fear, etc. Negativity makes your body tense, and inhibits all proper functioning. If you are under stress all the time, try to let it go during meals. This is a special time to nourish yourself on many levels.

(4) When you are ready to eat, take a few moments, center your-self, put all your cares aside, and allow yourself this time to relax and enjoy your meal.

(5) Consume foods and water as close to room temperature as possible. Extremes of hot or cold are a shock to the system, and can inhibit the production of digestive enzymes.

(6) Try not to slouch or wear tight clothing while you eat, as this can inhibit proper digestion.

(7) Don't wash your food down with water. Many people find they digest better if they do not take any liquids with meals.

If you are thirsty while you eat, chew and swallow your food first, then sip your water.

(8) Chew extremely well! It is in the chewing process that digestion begins. Chewing not only breaks food down, but stimulates the production of digestive enzymes.

(9) Undereat: Eat until you're satisfied, but not stuffed. This is essential for good health.

20

Basic Food Preparation

An unexpected bonus which many people experience when they switch to vital foods is the joy in the preparation itself. It is a touch with nature that is especially rare in city life, a way of making contact with the earth and its nourishing life force.

As you are becoming accustomed to new, healthier forms of food preparation, it may at first seem more complicated and time consuming than the methods you have been using. Be patient. This is a learning experience, and it always takes time at first to learn new ways of food preparation. Soon you will be amazed at how much simpler and more delicious healthy eating is.

Remember that in preparing quality meals, you are choosing increased health and vitality for you and your family.

A good health-maintenance program includes stress-free food preparation. This means (1) fast and easy preparation; and, (2) preserving the nutrients in your foods during the preparation.

FAST AND EASY FOOD PREPARATION

There are many ways to cut down on the time and energy it takes to prepare meals:

88

- Arrange your kitchen well.

- Purchase time-saving equipment and utensils.

- Keep in mind an over-all food plan.

- Have basic staples on hand. Include foods that cook quickly, such as rolled oats, whole grain noodles, kasha, fish, eggs, etc. Also have on hand staples that add flavor or texture to last minute cooking, such as garlic, onions, ginger, miso, tahini, kuzu, soup bouillons, etc. Also include some root vegetables, which may take longer to cook, but keep well and may save you a trip to the vegetable market.

- Keep some pre-prepared foods in the refrigerator or freezer to be ready to use in a variety of ways. For example, have on hand spreads, dips or dressings, sprouts, "sunburgers," lentil walnut burgers, cooked brown rice, cooked beans, cooked chicken, sauerkraut, washed and cut leafy greens and vegetables (although this is generally not advised, since washing and cutting results in a loss of nutrients).

- Use recipes that are easy and quick. The recipes in this book are very easy, but some are faster than others.

- Learn fast-cooking techniques, such as those which follow. (Note that these techniques are described more fully in each recipe section.)

FAST-COOKING TECHNIQUES

Most people find that using specific recipes requires more planning and shopping ahead, organization and time than they can afford.

It is simpler to refer to recipes for ideas, and then create a meal with ingredients that are on hand, easy to find, and that fit one's particular tastes and nutritional requirements. Learning a few fast-cooking techniques such as the following gives you this freedom.

The skeleton of a technique allows for more variety and creativity without excessive shopping and planning ahead.

NUT MILKS

Blend ground nuts and seeds, or nut/seed butter, such as tahini or almond butter, with water. Add pure sweeteners, flavorings or other ingredients. (See "Nut Milks," pp. 141–144.)

BASIC SOUP

Add to a broth any of the following in any combination: lightly steamed vegetables, cooked chicken or fish, cooked grains, noodles or beans, chopped parsley, chopped tomatoes. (See "Soups," p. 158.)

BLENDED SOUPS

Raw or lightly cooked vegetables, cooked beans or grains can be blended with hot or cold water or broth, plus spices, to make wonderful soups. (See p. 162.)

BLENDED CEREALS

Left over grains, such as rice, millet or barley, can be blended with hot water or nut milk and seasonings for a quick, hearty breakfast. (See p. 124.)

BLENDED SAUCES

Cooked grains or beans can be blended with hot water and spices, miso or tahini for a quick sauce. (See p. 193.)

BLENDED DRESSINGS

Raw vegetables can be blended with olive oil, lemon juice or apple cider vinegar and spices for a quick dressing. (See p. 186.)

GRAIN PILAF

Grains, nuts and seeds and lentils or split peas can be cooked in any combination in a broth, adding vegetables in the last couple of minutes of cooking. (See p. 231.)

MEAL-IN-ONE SAUTÉ

Lightly sauté on a low heat in olive oil or butter with any spices, any of the following in any combination: cooked grains, beans or pasta, lightly steamed or raw vegetables, cooked chicken or fish. Add ground nuts and seeds and a quick sauce.

QUICK STEAM SOUP OR MEAL IN A POT

Soups or whole meals can be created by steaming ingredients over a broth. (Other foods, such as pasta or fish, can meanwhile be cooking in the broth under the steamer.) For a soup, add the steamed ingredients to the broth. For a meal, separate the ingredients from the broth. For delicious examples, refer to Create-A-Soup, p. 164, and Create-A-Meal, p. 209.

SIMPLE SALAD

Mix raw or lightly steamed vegetables with cooked chicken, cooked beans, cooked pasta or cooked grains. Top with a dressing.

PREPARING FOOD TO PRESERVE NUTRIENTS

Foods should be prepared as close to eating time as possible. The longer you wait to eat foods after they have been washed, sliced and cooked, the more nutrients will have been lost.

To preserve nutrients and fiber in foods, prepare foods with as little heat as is reasonable for that particular food. Enzyme destruction begins at 130°. Also with high heat cooking, proteins become more difficult to digest or less available to the body, many vitamins and minerals are lost and fiber becomes less well utilized.

Never fry foods on high heat, since oils can become toxic at high heat, and fried, barbecued fats are carcinogenic (cancer causing). Use low heat when sautéeing. Use olive oil, canola oil, or butter for cooking, since it takes a higher heat for those oils to become toxic than for other oils.

Digestibility of fats is reduced when they are cooked beyond 250°.

You will note that not all the recipes in this book adhere strictly to low heat cooking. This takes into consideration transition cooking. For example, someone who has never before cooked brown rice will probably be more at ease cooking it the fast higher heat way (although the low heat cooking technique is also given). Many other recipes, although not as full of vitality as the low heat or raw food recipes presented in this book, are still delicious introductions to healthful eating.

SECTION III

RECIPES

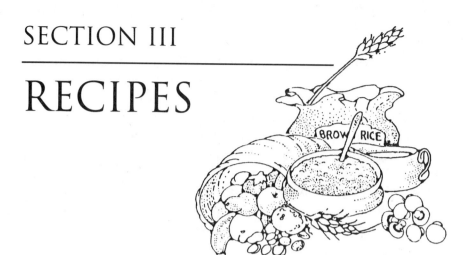

IMPORTANT NOTES

In reading recipes, please note the following guidelines:

- Use the purest of foods whenever possible:

    Oils: raw, cold pressed. For olive, use raw green or virgin olive oil
    Eggs: organic
    Chicken: organically raised, free-range
    Butter: unsalted; raw, if possible
    Honey: raw, unfiltered, organic
    Molasses: unsulphured
    Maple syrup: pure, unpasteurized
    Carob powder: raw, unsweetened
    Dried fruit: unsulphured, untreated
    Soy sauce: Use those with no toxic additives, such as MSG. Use
        wheat-free, if allergic to wheat. The wheat-free soy sauce often
        has a stronger taste, so you may need to use less than indicated.
    Apple cider vinegar: unpasteurized, organically made
    Water: spring; or distilled, if recommended by a nutrition con-
        sultant or doctor
    Vanilla extract: pure
    Baking powder: aluminum free
    Tofu: made without toxic additives

- Cook with olive oil, canola oil, or butter. For salads use cold pressed olive, sesame, sunflower, avocado, almond, flax, walnut or soy. "Sauté" means lightly stirring on a low heat.
- When using cayenne pepper, add it after cooking. High heat kills some of the valuable nutrients. When used raw, it is said to have strengthening properties. It is hot tasting, so add it gradually.

ABBREVIATIONS OF MEASUREMENTS

AMERICAN	METRIC
tsp. = teaspoon(s)	g. = gram(s)
Tbl.= Tablespoon(s)	L. = Liter(s)
c. = cup(s)	mL.= milliliter(s)
oz. = ounce(s)	
pt. = pint(s)	
qt. = quart(s)	
gal. = gallon(s)	
lb. = pound(s)	

AMERICAN AND METRIC EQUIVALENTS

AMERICAN	METRIC

Liquid Volume Equivalents

AMERICAN	METRIC
⅕ tsp.	1 milliliter
1 tsp.	5 milliliters
1 fluid ounce	30 milliliters
1 cup (8 oz.)	250 milliliters
1 pint (2 cups)	500 milliliters
1 quart (2 pints)	1 liter
1 gallon (4 qts.)	4 liters

Weight Equivalents

AMERICAN	METRIC
1 ounce	30 grams, or 16 drams
1 pound (16 oz.)	454 grams
2 pounds	1 kilogram

LIQUID VOLUME EQUIVALENTS

Tsp.	Tbl.	Fluid oz.	Cups	Pints	Quarts	Gallons	Metric
1/5 tsp.							= 1 mL
1 tsp.	= 1/3 Tbl.	= 60 drops					= 5 mL
3 tsp.	= 1 Tbl.						= 15 mL
6 tsp.	= 2 Tbl.	= 1 oz.					= 30 mL
12 tsp.	= 4 Tbl.	= 2 oz.	= 1/4 c.				
16 tsp.	= 5 1/3 Tbl. or 5 Tbl. + 1 tsp.	= 2 2/3 oz.	= 1/3 c.				
18 tsp.	= 6 Tbl.	= 3 oz.	= 3/8 c. or 1/4 c. + 2 Tbl.				
24 tsp.	= 8 Tbl.	= 4 oz.	= 1/2 c.				
26 tsp.	= 10 Tbl.	= 5 oz.	= 5/8 c. or 1/2 c. + 2 Tbl.				
36 tsp.	= 12 Tbl.	= 6 oz.	= 3/4 c.				
42 tsp.	= 14 Tbl.	= 7 oz.	= 7/8 c. or 3/4 c. + 2 Tbl.				
48 tsp.	= 16 Tbl.	= 8 oz.	= 1 c.	= 1/2 pt.			= 240 mL
96 tsp.	= 32 Tbl.	= 16 oz.	= 2 c.	= 1 pt.			= 480 mL
192 tsp.	= 64 Tbl.	= 32 oz.	= 4 c.	= 2 pt	= 1 qt.		= 1 liter
768 tsp.	= 256 Tbl.	= 128 oz.	= 16 c.	= 4 pt.	= 2 qt.	= 1 gal.	= 4 liters

COMMON FOOD EQUIVALENTS

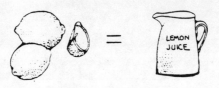

Almonds, unblanched, whole	1 c.	= 6 oz.
unblanched, ground	2⅔ c.	= 1 lb.
unblanched, slivered	5⅔ c.	= 1 lb.
blanched, whole	1 c.	= 5 ⅓ oz.
unblanched, whole	20 nuts	= 1 oz.
		= 4 Tbl. meal
Apples: fresh, peeled, chopped	5–6 c.	= 2 lbs. whole
dried, chopped, packed,	1 c.	= 4 ½ oz.
Apricots, dried	3 c.	= 1 lb.
cooked, drained	3 c.	= 1 lb.
Bananas, 3–4 medium sized, whole		= 1 lb.
mashed		= 2 c.
Barley	3 c.	= 1 lb.
	1c.	= 3½ c. cooked
Beans, uncooked, in general	2 c.	= 1 lb.
		= 6 c. cooked
Bean sprouts	¾ c.	= 15 oz.
Blueberries, whole	3 c.	= 1 pint
Bran	4 c.	= ½ lb.
Brown rice	2½ c.	= 1 lb.
	⅓ c.	= 1 c. cooked
Buckwheat	1 c.	= 4 c. cooked
Bulgur	4 c.	= 1⅓ lb.
Butter	1 stick	= 8 Tbl.
		= ½ c.
	4 sticks	= 2 c.
		= 1 lb.
Carrot, 6–7, sliced	3 c.	= 1 lb.
Celery, 2 medium sized or 1 large stalk		= 1 c. chopped
Cheese, fresh grated	5 c.	= 1 lb.
Cottage cheese	1 c.	= ½ lb.
Coconut, fine grated	3½ oz.	= 1 c.
shredded	5 c.	= 1 lb.

Cornmeal	3 c.	= 1 lb.
	1 c.	= 4 c. cooked
Currants, dried	2 c.	= 10 oz.
Dates, pitted	2½ c.	= 1 lb.
	18 dates	= ⅓ c.
Eggs, large	5	= about 1 c.
medium	6	= about 1 c.
small	7	= about 1 c.
egg whites	8–10	= 1 c.
egg yolks	12–14	= 1 c.
Flour	4 c.	= 1 lb.
Herbs, dried	1 tsp.	= 1 Tbl. fresh
Honey	1½ c.	= 1 lb.
Lemon	1	= 2–3 Tbl. juice
		= 2 tsp. rind
	1 tsp. juice	= ½ tsp. vinegar
Lime	1	= 1½ to 2 Tbl. juice
Molasses	1 c.	= 13 oz.
Mushrooms, sliced	1 c.	= ¼ lb.
Noodles, uncooked	1 lb.	= 7 c. cooked
Nuts, in the shell:		
almonds, walnuts	1½ c.	= 1 lb.
peanuts, pecans	2¼ c.	= 1 lb.
Nuts, shelled	1 c.	= 1 cup ground
pecans	2 c.	= 7½ oz.
	6 c.	= 1½ lb.
Oats, rolled	4 ¾ c.	= 1lb.
Onion, 1 large chopped		= 1 c.
Orange, 1 medium		= 7 Tbl. juice
		= 2½ Tbl. rind
Pepper, fresh green or red bell, chopped		= 1 c.
Pineapple, fresh, skinned, chopped	2 c.	= 1 lb.
Potatoes, raw, unpeeled	1 lb.	= 2 c. mashed
		= 3 c. chopped
Powdered milk	3 c.	= ½ lb.
Prunes, pitted	2¼ c.	= 1 lb.
cooked, drained	2 c.	= 1 lb.
Raisins, seeded, whole	3¼ c.	= 1 lb.
Scallion, 2 medium sized, chopped		= ¼ c.

Common Food Equivalents, cont.

Sesame seeds, hulled	4 c.	= 1 lb.
Sunflower seeds, hulled	4 c.	= 1 lb.
Tofu	2 c.	= 1 lb.
Tomatoes, 2 large chopped	3–4 c.	= 1 lb.
Water	2 c.	= 1 lb.
Wheat germ	2¼ c.	= ½ lb.
Winter squash, cooked	2 c.	= 2 lb.
Yeast, dry	4 Tbl.	= 1 oz.
Yogurt	2¼ c.	= 1 lb.
Zucchini, sliced	3½ c.	= 1 lb.

Sprouts

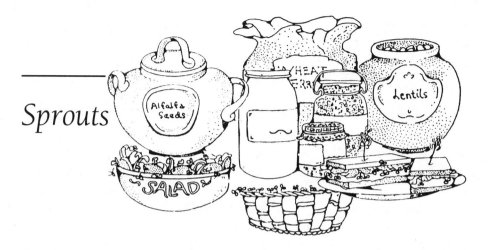

Sprouts are, very simply, a sprouted seed, bean or grain. They are the most vital and nourishing of all foods.

Sprouts are high in essential nutrients, are a good source of dietary fiber, low in calories, inexpensive and easy to prepare. Depending on the sprout, they contain varying amounts of vitamins A, B complex, C, D, E and K, factors G and U, and minerals such as calcium, magnesium, phosphorus, chlorine, potassium, iron, zinc and silicon.

Many sprouts contain all eight essential amino acids, which means that they are a good source of protein. The net protein utilized can be increased by combining certain sprouts, such as mung and lentil, at the same meal.

Sprouting increases the nutrient value of a seed. Vitamins C, B and E increase 10% to 30%, and the amount of protein can increase up to 1200%.

Sprouting also predigests the protein, making it more easily digested and assimilated, and breaks down the starch molecules into simple sugars, making sprouts a good energy food.

Sprouts can be added to any dish, such as sandwiches, salads, omelettes, cereals, breads, blender drinks, sauces, etc. It is best to cook sprouts grown from legumes and seeds (except buckwheat and sunflower seeds) to neutralize naturally-occuring toxins in the seeds and legumes.

HOW TO SPROUT

A seed holds within it the blueprint of life—all necessary elements for normal health and growth. Add to it water, air and sunshine, and a sprout will burst forth.

Sprouts are available in any health food store and in many super-markets. They are also fun to grow at home. It's easy to do, very inexpensive, and a great thrill to watch the little seeds grow into beautiful, delicious salad greens.

Children enjoy growing sprouts, and love to eat them, too. This is a great way to introduce them to the miracle of growing things, to have fun doing it, and to eat something super-packed with nutrition.

A variety of different types of seeds, beans or grains can be sprouted. If you have never sprouted before, try alfalfa for an easy beginning. Use seeds which have not been sprayed with chemicals. Purchase them at the health food store.

Three good ways to sprout will be described in the pages that follow:

(1) The traditional "jar" method, useful for sprouting seeds, beans or grains;
(2) The "basket" method, devised by Steve Meyerowitz ("Sproutman"). This method is best suited to sprouting seeds, such as alfalfa, fenugreek, clover and radish. It is not as suitable for sprouting grains or beans.
(3) The "bag" method, also devised by Sproutman, is great for sprouting grains and beans, but is not as suitable for seeds.

With the "jar" method, the seed, bean or grain is soaked and sprouted in the jar. With the "basket" method, the soaked seeds are transferred to a basket where they "root" themselves to the weave of the basket and grow straight toward the light. With the "bag" method, grains or beans are soaked and grown in a flaxseed bag.

When you begin sprouting, you will be amazed at how few seeds you need to produce a quantity of sprouts. They expand at least eight times their present size, so be sure the jar or bag is large enough to accomodate the increase, and that you do not use too many seeds.

For alfalfa seeds, two tablespoons for a quart size jar is good. If you use the basket method, use three tablespoons for a six inch basket, four tablespoons for an eight inch basket or five tablespoons for a nine inch basket. One to ten cups of grains or beans can be sprouted in the flaxseed bag, depending on the size of the bag.

When you soak the seeds, use spring water, as the seeds will absorb the water. It is not as important to use spring water for rinsing. Never use hot water, as it will sterilize the seeds and cause them to rot.

The time it takes for a sprout to reach maturity depends on the type of seed, the temperature of the weather, and the humidity. When it is hot, rinse more frequently to cool the seeds and to prevent mold.

Sprouts are generally ready when they are between one quarter and one and one half inches long. The sprout is past its peak when the second leaf system begins. Alfalfa sprouts are best at one inch long, and grain sprouts are ready when the length of the sprout equals the length of the grain. Refer to the "Sprouting Chart" for average time of maturation for each seed, bean or grain.

Sprouts will generally last as many days as it took for them to grow. For example, if the alfalfa sprouts took seven days to grow, they will last seven days.

Keep matured sprouts in the refrigerator. (The cold will slow down the growth of the sprouts, but won't stop it altogether.)

If you use the "jar" method, store the sprouts in a large glass jar or bowl, securely covered with cheesecloth and tipped at an angle so that any excess moisture can drain out.

If you use the "basket" method, you can put the basket with the sprouts and plastic all together in the refrigerator.

If you use the "bag" method, keep the bag, with the sprouts in it, in the refrigerator and rinse it once every other day.

SPROUTING INGREDIENTS & EQUIPMENT

For both the "jar" and the "basket" method, you will need:

(1) Your choice of seeds, beans or grains. (For simplicity in giving directions, I am illustrating with alfalfa seeds.)
(2) One or two wide mouthed jars, such as a mason jar, each 1 or 2 quart size.
(3) Cheese cloth or nylon mesh to cover the mouth of the jar.
(4) One or two rubber bands to secure the cheese cloth or mesh.

For the "basket" method, you will also need:

(5) An untreated straw basket (no shellac, please!) nine inches wide, and two and a half inches deep. Use one with a "tea-strainer" weave, which can usually be found at a houseware or oriental gift store.
(6) A plastic bag which fits over the basket and is strong enough not to "flop" onto the sprouts. The bag will create a "green house" effect. The plastic, unlike glass, will allow the sun's ultraviolet rays to shine through the sprouts. Ultraviolet rays are important for good health of the sprouts, and to kill any fungus.
(7) A gentle spray attachment for your faucet for rinsing the sprouts in the basket without disturbing their growth.

Don't be discouraged by the additional equipment required for the "basket" method. They are a one-time purchase, and well worth the advantages.

For the "bag" method, you will need:
One or several flaxseed bags, 100% pure—no chemicals added. Complete sprouting supplies can be ordered from The Sprout House, P.O. Box 1100, Great Barrington, MA 01230.

DIRECTIONS FOR SPROUTING

THE JAR METHOD

For Seeds, Beans or Grains

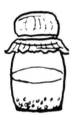 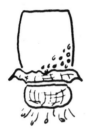 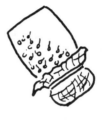 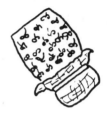

1. SOAK about 1 Tbl. alfalfa seeds for 4 hrs.

2. DRAIN off water.

3. Set Jar at 45% angle. Rinse twice per day.

4. Sprouts are ready in about 4 days. Refrigerate.

(1) Put one or two tablespoons of the selected seeds (or one cup of grains or beans) into the jar. Cover with the mesh or cheesecloth, and secure with a rubber band.

(2) Rinse the seeds several times, then fill the jar half way with lukewarm water, preferably spring water.

(3) Put the jar in a dark place, such as a cupboard. Let it soak overnight, or for the number of hours suggested on the sprouting chart.

(4) After the soak time, drain off the excess water. Rinse the seeds thoroughly with lukewarm water, again draining off excess water.

(5) Rest the jar in a saucer or dish rack, open end down, at a 45 degree angle so that excess water can drain off and the sprouts can breathe. (See drawing #3.)

Be sure the mesh at the jar opening is not covered by sprouts or hulls, and that air is free to contact the sprouts. Occasionally you may need to remove the mesh and scoop off the hulls which often cling to the mesh.

Hulls will automatically separate from the seeds as they sprout. They can create rot, which spreads quickly and can spoil a whole batch of sprouts.

(6) Thoroughly rinse and drain the sprouts two to three times a day until they are ready to eat—usually three to five days. Don't let the seeds dry out. Keep them moist, but not too wet.

(7) After about three days, put vegetable sprouts, such as alfalfa, clover and radish sprouts, in the light to let them "green," which means that chlorophyll, so important for good health, is manufactured. (Bean and grain sprouts do not need to be "greened.")

To help prevent mold caused by rotting hulls, occasionally remove the hulls in the following way (especially before "greening" or refrigerating sprouts):

Put the sprouts in a large bowl of water. Swish them around gently. Some hulls will float to the top and some hulls will sink to the bottom. Scoop off the hulls that are on the surface of the water. Then remove the sprouts, being careful not to stir up the hulls at the bottom of the bowl.

THE BASKET METHOD

For seeds

To sprout in a basket, follow the "jar" method and directions for steps 1–4. Use three to five tablespoons of seeds, depending on the size of your basket. Then continue with the following steps:

(5) Pour the soaked seeds into your basket. Tip the basket at an angle for a few minutes to drain off any excess water. You can lean the basket on a towel.

(6) Put the basket of seeds into a plastic bag and tuck the bag loosely underneath, so that you have created a "greenhouse" effect, allowing a bubble of trapped air.

(7) Rinse the seeds twice a day, gently but thoroughly, for a half a minute. Use a spray or shower adaptor, being careful not to disturb the root development. (The sprouts will anchor themselves by their roots to the weave of the basket.) Drain the basket well.

(8) When the hulls pop off and fall into the basket, rinse them off by immersing the basket in a basin of water. "Massage" the sprouts. The hulls will float up.

   After a few days, when the roots are securely anchored, put the basket upside down in the water. Again, gently "massage" the sprouts, and the hulls will drop off.

(9) When the top layers of sprouts are mature, gently pull them out with your fingers, being careful not to disturb the young sprouts underneath. Give this new generation a day or two and they will green up and grow to maturity. After you pluck them, there will be a third generation, and perhaps even a fourth.

THE BAG METHOD

For grains and beans

(1) Put about one cup grains or beans in a flaxseed bag. Soak the bag and seeds in pure water for eight to 12 hours.

(2) Hang the bag up so it will drain.

(3) Rinse the bag twice a day in cold water. Massage the bag a little while rinsing, to help keep the sprouts from rooting themselves to the bag.

(4) The sprouts will be mature in three to five days. Refrigerate them, rinsing them once every other day.

ADVANTAGES OF THE VARIOUS METHODS

THE JAR METHOD

The advantage in the jar method is that beans and grains, as well as seeds, can be sprouted in the jar.

THE BASKET METHOD

For sprouting seeds, the basket method has several advantages over the jar method:

(1) The basket allows for vertical growth of these miniature vegetables. Greater surface area is exposed to the light, allowing for greater development of chlorophyll.
(2) Sprouts are generally longer and healthier.
(3) The mature sprouts can be harvested before the immature sprouts, so you can have three to five generations of sprouts. In other words, you will have a greater yield of mature, green sprouts (12 to 15 times their volume, compared with seven to eight times their volume when using a jar).
(4) It is easier to clean hulls off the sprouting seeds than with the jar method.
(5) There is less chance for spoilage.

THE BAG METHOD

For sprouting grains or beans, the bag method has several advantages over the jar method:

(1) The bags drain well, allowing the seeds to breathe freely.
(2) Flax fiber, which is the material of the bag, absorbs moisture,

yet drains perfectly and maintains its coolness. For this reason, sprouts can be watered with a low risk of spoilage.

(3) Flax fiber is resistant to tearing, is light weight, easily transported, and takes up little space.

(4) The method of soaking and rinsing is simpler than with the jar method.

CHART FOR SPROUTING

SEED	SOAKING (Hours)	RINSING Times/day	READY IN (Days).
Aduki	8–12	3	3–5
Alfalfa	5–8	2–3	3–6
Chickpeas	8–15	4	3–4
Corn	8–15	3	2–3
Fava beans**	8–12	3	3–4
Fenugreek	6–8	3	3–4
Lentils	8–12	3	2–3
Millet	5–8	3	3–4
Mung beans	8–12	4	5–6
Oats	5–8	2	3–4
Peas	8–15	2	3–5
Radishes	5–8	2	3–5
Red clover	5–8	4	5–7
Rye	8–12	3	2–3
Soybeans	15–24	4	3–4
Sunflower seeds	8	2	1
Wheat	8–15	2	2–3

**The same applies to all beans: black, white, haricot, kidney, lima, navy, pinto, and red beans, etc.

From "Recipes for Life" by Dr. Ann Wigmore.
Reprinted with permission of Hippocrates World Health Organization.

Breads & Muffins

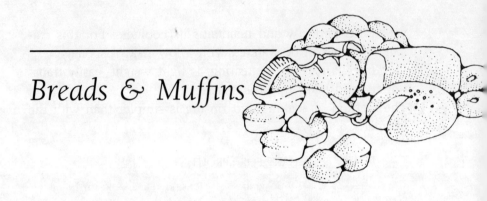

There are many marvelous recipe books that you can consult for baking a variety of delicious breads. The emphasis here is on breads that are easy to make and primarily wheat-free.

Essene bread is a thick, chewy bread, made from sprouted grains and baked on a low heat. Because it is nearly raw, it is especially high in nutrients and vitality.

The Quick 2-Slice Bread Recipe was created out of the dilemma of wanting a slice of wheat-free bread for a meal or two, but not wanting to buy a whole loaf, or to take the time to bake one. The recipe creates two slices of delicious bread that are done in 15 minutes and are sturdy enough to top with a spread and sprouts.

To help avoid an allergy to wheat, vary your grains as much as possible.

Since all flour should be refrigerated, warm the amount of flour you need before using it for about 15 minutes in a low oven (150°). If you are using wheat germ, which is also refrigerated, warm that, too.

BREAD RECIPES

ESSENE BREAD

This bread is raw, made from sprouted grains.
   Use any of the following grains:

wheat	rye
unhulled barley	whole oats
triticale	

Soak 1½ c. grain overnight in 4 c. water.
   In the morning, drain the water and let the grains sprout for 36 hours or more, until their "tails" measure about ⅛ inch long. During this time, rinse them 2–3 times a day.
   Grind the sprouts in a hand grinder, seed processor, or Champion juicer.
   Knead the sticky mixture until it is a doughlike consistency and it begins to hold shape.

Add any flavorings you like, such as:

chopped dates	sunflower seeds
chia seeds	onion
sesame seeds	chives
caraway seeds	raisins
garlic	cumin
dill seeds	

Shape into loaves or patties. Lightly oil the surface of the dough and place on a well-oiled pan.
   Put the pan in a low heat oven—150°, or on a warm spot of a wood stove, or in the summer sun. The bread is done when there is a thin crust on the outside, and the inside is soft and moist, but not sticky. (Approximately 6 to 8 hours of drying.)
   Note that this bread will be heavier than those to which you are accustomed.

EVA'S BREAD

3 c. rye or whole wheat flour	2 Tbl. honey
1 Tbl. baking powder	2 eggs or 1 egg + 2 egg whites
1½ c. water	

Preheat the oven to 350°.

Thoroughly mix the flour and baking powder. Blend the water, honey and eggs in a blender, then pour the mixture over the dry ingredients. Mix well, using quick strokes. Place in a lightly oiled or buttered loaf pan and bake at 350° for about 55 minutes, or until the top is well browned. Let it cool before slicing.

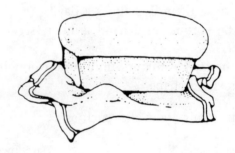

Variations:

Use any whole grain flour, such as millet, oat, barley, etc., or any combination of flours. (You may need to add more flour or water to get the same dough consistency.)

Add to the bread dough nuts or seeds, such as 2–3 tsp. caraway, sesame or sunflower seeds, or add raisins, chives, sliced onion or herbs. For a spice bread add more honey and/or molasses, plus cinnamon, ginger and allspice.

To make rolls, use 2 c. flour, 1 Tbl. baking powder, 2 eggs, 2 Tbl. honey and 1 c. water. Bake in muffin tins at 325° for 30–35 minutes, until the tops are golden brown. This makes 8 muffins.

Experiment to your heart's content.

The bread recipe is from *The Good Book Cookbook* by Eva Graf and Mitch Seagrave.

QUICK 2–SLICE BREAD

If you have some left-over cereal, and wish you had a slice of bread, create two slices in your toaster oven in a matter of minutes.

Ingredients

½ c. buckwheat porridge or creamy rice cereal, or corn-meal cereal cooked with al-mond milk	¼ c. almonds 1 egg

Grind the almonds in a blender. If you want some chunks of nuts in the bread, don't completely pulverize the nuts.

Leave the ground nuts in the blender. Add to the blender the cooked grain and one egg. Blend well.

Lightly grease your toaster oven pan. Spoon two large circles, or squares of the mixture onto the pan. Spread them out slightly so that they are a little flat, like bread.

Bake at 400° 15 minutes for buckwheat bread, or ½ hour for corn or rice bread.

The buckwheat bread is delicious with 1 tsp. caraway seeds added to the batter. Top the bread with miso/tahini spread and alfalfa sprouts.

Top the cornmeal bread with butter and honey.

Note: For a low-heat baking method, preheat the toaster oven to 450°. Put the bread in the oven. Turn the heat off. Let sit overnight.

MILLET BANANA BREAD (*Makes 1 loaf*)

1 c. mashed bananas (about 2 bananas)

2 eggs, beaten or 1 egg plus 2 egg whites

¼ c. honey

¼ c. melted butter (½ stick) or "better butter" (see p. 36)

2 Tbl. non-fat plain yogurt (optional)

1 c. millet flour (purchased, or freshly ground in your nut-seed or grain grinder, or ex-coffee mill)

1 tsp. baking soda

½ c. chopped walnuts (optional)

Preheat the oven to 350°.

Mix the wet ingredients in one bowl, and the dry ingredients in another bowl. Combine them, then pour into a lightly greased 9x3x5" loaf pan.

Bake at 350° for 55–60 minutes.

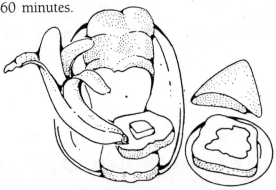

ZUCCHINI BREAD (*Makes 1 loaf*)

Preparation time: 35 minutes
Baking time: 45–55 minutes

2 eggs, beaten	1 tsp. baking soda
2 Tbl. plain yogurt	1½ c. whole wheat pastry flour
¾ c. honey	1½ tsp. ground cinnamon
¼ c. melted butter (½ stick)	½ c. chopped walnuts (optional)
1 c. grated zucchini (about 1 medium sized zucchini)	

Preheat the oven to 350°.

In a large bowl beat the eggs, then add the yogurt and mix well. Add the melted butter and honey and mix well, then add the grated zucchini and mix well.

In a separate bowl, mix the dry ingredients. Add the dry ingredients to the wet and mix well.

Lightly grease a 9x5x3" loaf pan. Pour the mixture into the pan and bake at 350° for 45–55 minutes. It's done when a toothpick comes out clean in the center and the edges are a medium brown. Gently remove and let cool on a wire rack.

Note: To make a *PUMPKIN SPICE BREAD,* use this same recipe with the following changes:

Use 1 cup steamed, mashed pumpkin in place of raw, grated zucchini.

In addition to the cinnamon, use ½ tsp. allspice, ⅛ tsp, nutmeg and ⅛ tsp. ginger. Bake at 350° for 55 minutes.

GINGERBREAD

½ c. rice flour
1 c. oat flour
2 tsp. baking powder
1 tsp. ground cinnamon
1 tsp. ground ginger
¼ tsp. ground cloves
3 egg yolks

½ c. molasses
¾ c. honey
½ c. melted butter or "better butter" (see p. 36)
¼ c. water
3 egg whites

Preheat the oven to 350°.

Mix the flours, baking powder and spices in a large bowl.

In a medium sized bowl, beat the egg yolks. Add the melted butter, honey, molasses and water. Stir till well mixed.

Add the liquid ingredients to the dry, and stir till well blended.

In a medium sized bowl, beat the egg whites until they form soft peaks.

Fold the egg whites gently into the batter.

Pour into a lightly greased 8" baking pan.

Bake at 350° for 40–45 minutes, or until done. Gently remove the bread from the pan and let cool on a wire rack.

Top with pure whipped cream. (Sweetener is not necessary, although if you like, you could add a small amount of honey.)

Or, top with lemon frosting, non-fat vanilla yogurt or kefir cheese.

CORN MUFFINS (*Makes 16 muffins*)

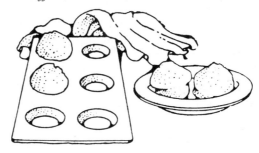

Preheat the oven to 425°, and lightly grease a 16 muffin tin.

Beat together in a bowl, or blend in a blender the following wet ingredients:

3 eggs	3 Tbl. honey
6 Tbl. melted butter	1¾ c. water

Note: Before the butter has cooled, add the honey to it and stir until the honey dissolves. Add the water to this mixture to cool it off before adding it to the eggs. Otherwise, the hot butter may cook the eggs.

In a large bowl, mix together the following dry ingredients:

3 c. cornmeal
1 Tbl. baking powder (aluminum-free)
optional: ½ tsp. sea salt

Add the wet ingredients to the dry, and stir till well mixed. Scoop or ladle the batter from the bottom of the mixing bowl (in case the cornmeal settles) and pour into each muffin mold, leaving some room for the dough to rise. Bake for 20 minutes at 425°, or until the muffins are golden brown.

APPLESAUCE MUFFINS (*Makes 8 muffins*)

¾ c. ground rolled oats (Grind 1 c. rolled oats in your blender.)
¾ c. brown rice flour
1 tsp. baking soda
3 Tbl. honey
¼ c. melted butter

1 egg yolk
½ tsp. orange extract
1 Tbl. grated organic orange peel
¾ c. unsweetened applesauce
½ c. currants
1 egg white

Preheat the oven to 400°.
Lightly grease an 8 cup muffin pan.

In a large mixing bowl, mix the ground rolled oats, brown rice flour and baking soda.

In a smaller bowl, beat the egg yolk. Add the honey, melted butter, orange extract and grated orange peel. Stir well till mixed. Add the applesauce and the currants, stirring till mixed.

Slowly add the liquid ingredients to the dry, stirring with quick strokes till combined.

Beat the egg white till it forms soft peaks. Gently fold the beaten egg white into the batter till well mixed.

Spoon the batter into the greased muffin tins, filling them two-thirds full.

Bake at 400° for 20–25 minutes till done. Remove the muffins from the tin and let cool on a wire rack.

Variation:

Omit the orange extract and grated orange peel. Add 1 tsp. cinnamon.

AMARANTH MUFFINS

1½ c. amaranth flour (grind amaranth till you have a flour)
1 tsp. baking soda
¼ tsp. cinnamon
2 egg yolks
3 Tbl. honey

2 Tbl. oil
1 c. soy milk
3 tsp. grated orange rind
¼ c. raisins
2 egg whites

Prepare a 12-cup muffin pan (2½" size) by brushing bottoms and sides with oil. Preheat oven to 375°.

Mix flour, baking soda and cinnamon in a medium size mixing bowl.

In a large mixing bowl, beat egg yolks till thick. Add honey, oil, soy milk, orange rind and raisins. Mix, then add flour mixture.

In a separate bowl, beat egg whites till stiff. Gently fold into batter.

Spoon mixture into muffin tins, filling ⅔ full.

Bake 30 minutes.

Cereals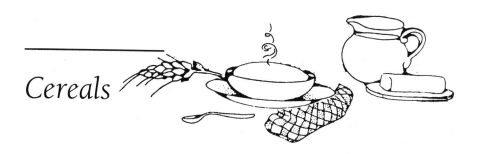

Cereals that are easy to prepare, delicious and well balanced proteins are a wonderful way to start a day and to sustain strength and energy for hours.

INGREDIENTS FOR CEREALS

WHOLE GRAINS

oats: rolled, steel-cut or sprouted.
millet: whole, freshly ground, sprouted.
barley: whole, freshly ground, roasted or flaked.
rice: whole, freshly ground.
rye: sprouted, flaked, freshly ground.
buckwheat: unroasted or roasted (kasha).
wheat: freshly ground, sprouted or flaked.
corn meal.

NUTS AND SEEDS

soaked, freshly ground or sprouted:

almonds	sunflower seeds
sesame seeds	pumpkin seeds
chia seeds	flax seeds
caraway seeds	walnuts

REHYDRATED (SOAKED) DRIED FRUIT

whole or chopped:

prunes	raisins
dates	figs
apricots	currants

FRESH FRUIT

bananas	peaches
berries	apples

OTHER OPTIONAL CEREAL INGREDIENTS

grated coconut	butter
honey	maple syrup
barley malt	molasses
soy sauce	cinnamon
tahini	miso

LIQUID BASES OR TOPPINGS FOR CEREALS

Water
Nut/seed milk, soy milk or grain water
Juice, such as apple juice

Cereals can be cooked in, or topped with these liquids.

GENERAL CEREAL COOKING TECHNIQUES

Cereals, as with any grains, should be cooked on low heat to preserve nutrients and vitality.

Cereals can be cooked in any of the following ways, depending on the type of grain:

1. *For rolled oats, buckwheat or sprouted grain:*
   Bring grain and liquid just to the boil, shut off the heat, cover the pot and let the grain cook in its own steam.
2. *For any cooked grain:*
   a. In a blender, blend cooked grain with hot liquid, or,
   b. Heat the cooked grain in a pot mixed with a liquid, then eat as is, or blend.
3. *For sprouted grain, whole or ground brown rice, millet, barley or rye:*
   a. Gently cook on the lowest possible heat, or,
   b. Soak the grain for 24 to 36 hours. Then, the night before eating the cereal, bring the grain close to the boil, shut off the heat, cover the pot and let the grain cook in its own steam.

HELPFUL CEREAL HINTS

TIME SAVING PREMIX

Mix any of the following cereal ingredients in any combination(s) and keep them in glass jars in the freezer (to avoid rancidity) till use:

nuts and seeds   grated coconut
dried fruit   whole grains
sprouted grain

FOR EASIER DIGESTIBILITY

Soak or grind the nut/seed mixture before adding to the cereal. Flax, sesame and chia, especially, should be ground since they are too small and hard to be chewed well.

Soak the dried fruit mixture over night, or add to the cereal before cooking.

FOR A MORE COMPLETE PROTEIN

Mix different kinds of grains, and add a variety of nuts and seeds to your cereals. For example, mix millet, wheatberries, buckwheat, and sesame, sunflower and flax seeds.

Or, use nut milk or soy milk to top your cereal, or as a cooking liquid.

FLAVOR CHANGER

Cook the cereal in nut milk instead of water. Use different kinds of nuts and seeds and, in a blender, blend different sweeteners and/or dried fruit in the nut milk.

CEREAL RECIPES

Cereal recipes are categorized by preparation time, since that is often an important consideration in the morning. The categories are as follows:

"SUPER QUICK CEREALS": These take 10 to 20 minutes.

"30 MINUTE CEREALS": These take between 30 and 45 minutes, although with some planning ahead they can take less time without sacrificing nutrition.

"THINK AHEAD CEREALS": These take some pre-preparation, but once that is done, are super quick and super delicious.

SUPER QUICK CEREALS

These take 10 to 20 minutes, including preparation and cooking time.

OATMEAL (*Makes 1 cup*)

½ c. rolled oats   1¼ c. water or nut milk
Optional: 1–2 Tbl. raisins and/or honey

Put the water or nut milk in a pot. Add the oats (and dried fruit). Bring the liquid close to a boil while stirring.

Turn the heat off, cover the pot, and let the oatmeal cook in its own steam till soft (about 10 minutes).

Eat as is, or add butter and/or soy or nut milk, or tahini and/or miso.

To make a creamy oatmeal, put the cooked oatmeal through the blender with hot water or nut milk.

BUCKWHEAT PORRIDGE (*Makes 1 cup*)

(Note: Buckwheat is not wheat. Those with wheat allergies can often tolerate buckwheat.)

½ c. buckwheat or kasha   ½ c. water
  (roasted buckwheat)

Put the buckwheat and water in a pot. Bring the water just to the boil. Turn off the heat. Stir the buckwheat with a fork. Cover the pot and let sit till soft (5–10 minutes). Top with nut milk, or butter and soy sauce. This makes a great side dish, as well.

Optional:

Add soaked dried fruit.

QUICK CREAM OF GRAIN CEREAL (*Makes 1 cup*)

2 versions:
  1. Grind nuts and seeds in a dry blender. Add about ¾ c. cooked grain (such as brown rice or millet) and ¼ c. hot water. Blend again. Add as much water as you like for the consistency desired.

(or)

  2. Warm cooked grain in a pot with almond or soy milk. Eat as is or blenderize.

For a less sweet taste that is delicious, try re-heating or blending the cooked grain in soy milk and a pinch of cinnamon. Or, in place of cinnamon, add a small amount of light miso when the cereal is ready to eat.

Note: Adding nuts and seeds, nut milk or soy milk to cereals not only enhances the flavor, but increases the utilizable protein.

30-MINUTE CEREALS

30 MINUTE CREAM OF GRAIN CEREAL (*Makes 1 c.*)

¼ c. freshly ground brown rice
   or millet
1 c. almond milk, sweetened

with honey or molasses, cinnamon, and pure vanilla extract.
¼ c. raisins

Put almond milk, ground grain and raisins in a pot. Bring just to the boiling point, stirring constantly, until the grain flour has absorbed the liquid. Turn off the heat and cover the pot.* Put the pot over a double boiler on a low simmer for 20–30 minutes.

* Note: For quicker cooking in the morning, prepare the grain up to this point the night before, soaking the grain and the raisins in the hot liquid overnight. In the morning, bring it close to the boil again, then put it over the double boiler for 10 to 15 minutes.

Optional:

Add sliced bananas and/or nut milk.

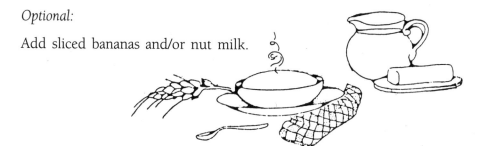

MILLET CEREAL (*Makes 1 cup*)

¼ c. millet   1 c. water or nut milk
Optional:
nuts/seeds or dried fruit

Put the water or nut milk (plus optional extras) in a pot. Bring just
to the boil, then turn heat down to the lowest possible setting. Cook
about 20 minutes, till soft. Eat as is, or with sliced bananas and
nut milk.

CORN MEAL CREAM CEREAL (*Makes 1½ c*)

(Takes about 45 minutes, including cooking)

1¼ c. almond milk   ¼ c. corn meal
1 tsp. molasses   ⅛ tsp. vanilla
¼–½ tsp. cinnamon   1 Tbl. raisins

Prepare the nut milk, blending into it the molasses, cinnamon and
vanilla.
Meanwhile, heat water in the bottom of a double boiler, leaving it
at a low simmer.

Put the nut milk in the top of the double boiler. Put that pot
directly over the burner and while bringing the nut milk close to a
boil, slowly pour in the corn meal (plus raisins) while stirring constantly with a wire whisk to avoid lumping.

When the almond milk has absorbed the corn meal, cover the
pot and put it over the bottom of the double boiler.

Let stand over the double boiler, which is still at a low simmer,
½ hour.

Brown Barley Cream Cereal (*Makes 1 cup*)

¼ c. barley	1 tsp. raw honey
¾ c. water	

Spread the barley kernels thinly in a frying pan. Brown them lightly, stirring constantly. (This procedure is not necessary, but makes a more delicious taste.)

Put the browned barley in a pot. Add the water. Bring just to the boiling point. Take the pot off of the heat. Cover and let stand 20 minutes.

If you like, blend the cooked barley, adding honey, barley malt, miso or molasses, etc. Top with nut milk.

THINK AHEAD CEREALS

These cereals take some thinking ahead and preparation, but are well worth it! (This could also include the super quick rice, millet and barley cream cereals since the grains must be cooked ahead of time.)

Sprouted Cereal: Wheat or Rye

1 ounce of dry seed produces about 1 cup of mature sprouts. Sprouts can expand to at least eight times their seed size.

To use sprouted grains as a cereal, mix them in any combination you like by themselves or with the quick-cook grains (such as rolled oats, rye flakes, buckwheat, etc.) Add freshly ground or soaked nuts and seeds, soaked dried fruit, etc. Top with nut milk.

THERMOS CEREAL

For any grain except wheat, which becomes too rubbery. The rolled or flaked cereals may also be too mushy cooked this way.

Use a one quart wide mouthed thermos. Add the grain and any other ingredients (nuts and seeds, dried fruit, etc.), then the required amount of nearly boiling liquid. (Do not fill water right up to the top. Allow at least one inch from the top.)

Screw the lid on tightly and let stand eight to 12 hours.

Grains can be put into the thermos whole or ground. If you like, blend the cooked cereal.

SUPER CEREAL

Step 1.

Put a mixture of grains in a large bowl or jar and add water 2½ times the volume of the grain. Let stand on the counter for 36 hours at room temperature.

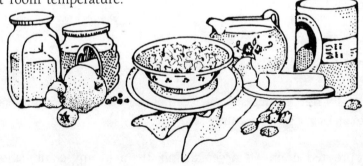

Step 2.

After the 36 hour soaking time, refrigerate. To keep it fresh and moist, cover the grain with water. This will keep for several days.

Step 3.

The night before you want the cereal, remove ½ to 1 cup of the mixture, leaving the remaining portion covered with water in the refrigerator.

Put the pre-soaked mixture in a pot, add any additional quick-cook grains, nuts and seeds, or dried fruit, plus an equal amount of water.

Bring the water just to the boil, shut the heat off, cover the pot, and let stand overnight.

Step 4.

The next morning, warm the mixture, and add to taste: honey or barley malt, butter and nut milk or soy milk.

Suggested grains to pre-soak:

brown rice	millet
wheatberries	whole rye

Add the night before

rye flakes	rolled oats	buckwheat
sunflower seeds	pumpkin seeds	almonds
dried fruit	shredded coconut	
ground flax and/or sesame seeds		

Note: All ingredients listed under "Add the night before" can be pre-mixed to taste and kept on hand in the freezer.

GOLDEN ROASTED GRANOLA (*Makes about 5 cups*)

¼ c. melted butter, canola oil, or "better butter" (see p. 36)

¼ c. honey or barley malt

1 tsp. vanilla extract

3 c. rolled oats

1 tsp. cinnamon

¼ c. hulled, ground sesame seeds

¾ c. dry roasted, unsalted soybeans

¾ c. chopped almonds, pecans or walnuts

¼ c. ground flax seeds

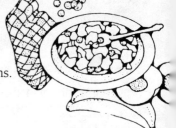

Optional:

1 c. shredded coconut or ¾ c. dates; 1 c. raisins.

Preheat oven to 250°.

Mix the butter, honey or barley malt, and vanilla. Mix the oats and cinnamon in another bowl. Pour the butter mixture over the oat mixture and mix well.

Lightly oil a flat pan. Thinly spread the mixture onto the pan.

Bake for 1 to 1½ hours, stirring occasionally, until the mixture is a light golden brown. (For lower-heat baking, preheat the oven to 300° the night before, then shut it off when you put the pan in, and leave it overnight.)

Remove the mixture from the oven, and add the nuts and seeds and any optional ingredients. Store in an airtight container in the refrigerator.

Note: The dry ingredients can be premixed and kept in jars in the freezer till use.

Pancakes

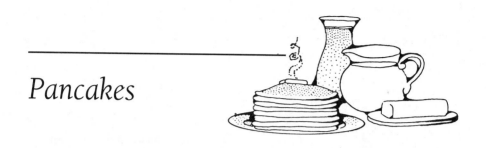

GENERAL PANCAKE COOKING HINTS

To test your griddle to see if it is the right heat, drop a little water on it. If the water bounces around, the griddle is the right heat. If the water just sits there, it is not hot enough. If the water quickly evaporates, the griddle is too hot.

Spoon the pancake batter onto the griddle from a height just above the pan. The pancake will be ready to turn when tiny air bubbles form (and before they pop). Usually the pancake will take half the cooking time on the other side, after it is turned.

To keep the pancakes warm, put them on a baking sheet in a low oven. Do not stack them right on top of each other, or they will get rubbery. Put a cloth between each one.

RECIPES

BUCKWHEAT PANCAKES (*about 2 dozen*)

1 c. buckwheat flour
½ c. brown rice flour
½ tsp. baking soda
1½ c. buttermilk

4 Tbl. melted butter, or canola oil
2 eggs, beaten

Combine the flours and the baking soda.

In a separate bowl, beat the eggs. Add the melted butter or oil and buttermilk.

Add the liquid ingredients to the dry, combining them well with quick strokes. Add water till you have a fairly runny batter. (About ⅓ to ½ c. water.)

CORNMEAL PANCAKES

1 c. yellow cornmeal
1¼ c. boiling water
½ c. brown rice flour
2 tsp. baking powder
1 egg yolk
½ c. almond milk (10 almonds
   ground, then blended with ½
   c. water and 2 tsp. honey.)

2 Tbl. melted butter or canola oil
1 egg white

Put the cornmeal in a large bowl. Slowly stir in the 1¼ c. boiling water till well combined. Let stand 10 minutes.

In a separate bowl, beat the egg yolk. Add the almond milk and butter or oil.

Combine the rice flour and baking powder, then add to the cornmeal.

Add the liquid ingredients and stir till well mixed.

Beat the egg white till it forms soft peaks. Gently fold the beaten egg white into the batter.

If necessary, add more water so that the batter is slightly runny.

PANCAKE VARIATIONS

Add to pancake batter any of the following:

chopped banana
blueberries
ground cinnamon

chopped walnuts
chopped apples

FOR PANCAKE TOPPINGS, SEE NEXT PAGE.

PANCAKE TOPPINGS

Pancakes are great topped with any of the following:

- pure maple syrup

- homemade mixtures, such as:
    honey + butter + cinnamon
    barley malt + butter + cinnamon
    molasses + butter + cinnamon
    tahini, barley malt, cinnamon, and water, mixed well to thin

- fresh fruit jam or marmalade, such as honey carrot marmalade or strawberry jam

- applesauce

- yogurt or kefir cheese

- silken tofu + banana + pineapple concentrate

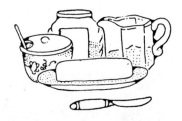

Eggs

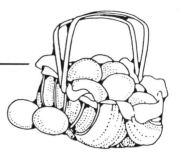

Soft boiling or poaching are the best ways to cook eggs, since over-cooked proteins are less utilizable by the body and are often difficult to digest.

SOFT BOILING

Put the egg(s) in a pot and cover with cool water. Bring the water close to a boil, then turn the heat off. Let the egg(s) cook in the steam water, covered, for 2–4 minutes, depending on how "runny" you like them.

OMELETTES

If you make omelettes, cook with a small amount of butter, canola oil or olive oil on the lowest possible heat, and do not over-cook.

Delicious omelette fillings:
plain yogurt + chopped scallion + alfalfa sprouts + sliced zucchini
cottage cheese + sliced avocado + chopped watercress leaves

SCRAMBLING AND FRYING

If you scramble or fry your eggs, do it in a small amount of butter, canola oil or olive oil on a low heat. Alfalfa sprouts are delicious added to scrambled eggs after cooking.

POACHING

Bring about 2 inches water in a fry pan to a low simmer below the boiling point. Add a drop of apple cider vinegar. (This helps hold the egg together.)

Crack one egg at a time, slipping it into the gently simmering water. If the white of the egg spreads too far, you can gently push it toward the yolk with a spatula. Simmer for 4 to 5 minutes, or remove the pan from the heat and let sit 8 minutes. Cook the egg till it holds, but is not hard.

Some people find that the egg will be less likely to spread if they make a whirlpool in the water with a spoon before adding the egg. Then slip the egg into the center of the well of the whirlpool.

If there are streamers of white after the egg is cooked, you can cut them off with scissors before serving.

If you have difficulty digesting proteins and starches together (poached eggs on toast), serve the egg over steamed broccoli or spinach. Put a small amount of butter and/or lemon juice on the vegetable before adding the egg.

Beverages

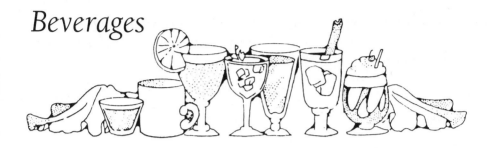

Fresh juices and blender drinks made from raw vegetables and fruits, nuts, seeds, and grains are perhaps the most delicious and enjoyable way to fill an undernourished body with a concentration of quickly and easily assimilated nutrients, while gently, but powerfully accelerating the process of detoxification and regeneration.

Juices and blender drinks are a great way to get a lot of variety in the diet.

Freshly juiced vegetables, greens and fruits can also be used effectively, under your doctor's care, to lose or gain weight, or to undertake a health-regaining juice fast.

Juices and blender drinks can also provide crucial nourishment to those with denture problems or extreme digestive stress.

In addition, when you have more fruits, vegetables and leafy greens than you can use in your recipes, they need not go to waste. Juice or blend them in any of the delicious combinations suggested in this recipe section.

BEVERAGE VARIETIES

Delicious and healthful beverages can be prepared quickly and easily with a juice extractor or a blender, depending on the recipe, and there is an almost unlimited variety.

NUT/SEED MILKS

Nut/Seed milks are "milky" liquids made by blending nuts and seeds, or nut/seed butters (such as tahini or almond butter), and water. They are a good source of easily assimilated protein, of B vitamins and other vitamins, minerals, oils and unsaturated fatty acids, and, best of all, they taste wonderful!

In a whole state, nuts and seeds can be difficult to chew, especially the smaller seeds, and are tempting to over-eat, a strain on the digestion and on body weight. With nut milks, the nuts and seeds are broken down to a more easily digested form, and, since they are measured out in the preparation, the temptation to over-indulge is eliminated.

Nut milks are a great substitute for cow's milk in any recipe, especially over cereal. They are non-mucus forming, rarely allergenic, and provide calcium and other minerals necessary for calcium absorption and utilization.

Nut milks are also a wonderful base for smoothies and for beverages that provide a breakfast in a glass. Simply blend the nut milk with fruit, such as a banana or an organic raw egg to create the effect you desire.

GRAIN WATER

For those who prefer not to have nuts and seeds or dairy, and/or need a large intake of minerals, grain water is an ideal solution.

It is delicious on cereals, as a snack, as a soup or sauce base, and is perfect for convalescing or denture problems. It is made by blending a small amount of cooked grain, such as barley, rice or millet with water.

Rejuvelac, or fermented grain water, made by soaking wheat or rye berries in water for 24–48 hours, is an excellent source of lactic acid (which feeds "friendly bacteria," so necessary for a healthy colon), and of enzymes, and vitamins E and B.

VEGETABLE COCKTAILS

Freshly juiced raw vegetables contain valuable vitamins, minerals, enzymes and natural sugars, and are easily digested since the cellulose has been removed. They can be prepared in many delicious combinations, according to taste preference and nutritional needs.

GREEN DRINKS

Green drinks are a great way to get lots of chlorophyll, which is one of our most powerful aids in balancing, cleansing and rebuilding a weak body. Use a variety of greens, such as watercress, parsley, romaine lettuce, etc.

Wheatgrass juice, the juice from the green grass grown from wheat berries, is possibly the best source of chlorophyll we have. SImply chew the grass and spit out the pulp, or juice it with a press-type juicer designed to extract juice from wheatgrass. (Drink very small amounts of wheatgrass juice at a time, as it is very strong—not more than 1/2–1 oz.)

Wheatgrass can be grown with the basket method of sprouting (p. 104) or can be purchased fresh or frozen in a health food store.

PINEAPPLE COCKTAILS

Pineapple juice combines well with vegetables and/or proteins, can aid the digestion, and has a gently cleansing action.

OTHER JUICED AND BLENDED FRUITS

Children, and the child in each of us, especially love fruit juices in homemade soft drinks, smoothies and shakes.

BEVERAGE RECIPES

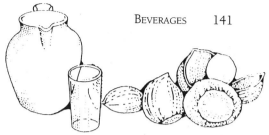

NUT/SEED MILKS

There are many variations on nut milks. Use your imagination and taste preferences to experiment.

Nut/Seed Choices

almond	sunflower	pumpkin
sesame	chia	flax

Keep your own special mixture of whole nuts and seeds in a glass jar in the freezer (to avoid rancidity) to grind when needed. They take only seconds to grind.

Note that the "butters" made from nuts and seeds, such as tahini (sesame seed butter), or almond butter, can also be blended with water to form nut milks.

Liquid Base Variations For Nut Milks

water	
pineapple juice	vegetable juice
grain water	soup bouillon

Nut Milk Blending Variations

1. Soak nuts and seeds of your choice overnight, then blend with the liquid.
2. Without soaking first:
   a. Grind the nuts and seeds in a dry blender, then add liquid, or,

  b. Put the nuts and seeds and liquid in the blender together,
     then blend.
3. Blend tahini or almond butter with water.

The method of grinding the nuts and seeds depends on the type
of blender—the strength and position of the blade. Find the method
that works best for you.

A nut/seed grinder (your ex-coffee mill) works best for smaller
seeds, such as sesame, flax, or chia. After grinding them, transfer
them to the blender to blend with the liquid.

A normal blender or Cuisinart will usually grind nuts and larger
seeds, and sometimes larger quantities of smaller seeds.

You may wish to strain the nut milk after blending, to remove
small particles, especially if you are feeding a small child.

Add to Nut Milks Any of the Following:

whey powder

brewers yeast

rice polishings

tahini

molasses

rice bran syrup

ground cloves

black cherry concentrate

unsweetened carob powder (a
  "chocolate" taste)

cafix (a "coffee" flavor)

vanilla or almond extract

fresh or soaked dried fruit

raw vegetables and/or
  leafy greens

soy powder

lemon juice

almond butter

barley malt

cinnamon

shredded coconut

wheat germ

tofu

bran

honey

maple syrup

nutmeg

NUT MILK RECIPES

ALMOND MILK (*Makes 1 cup*)

8–10 almonds	¾ c. water
⅛ tsp. vanilla	¼ tsp. honey

Grind the almonds in a dry blender, then add the water, vanilla and honey and blend well again. Strain, if necessary.

Optional:

Some people prefer to blanch the almonds first; that is, to remove the skins.

Blanching almonds:

   Bring some water to a boil, drop the almonds in the water, turn the heat off and let the almonds sit a minute or two. Break a tiny hole in the skin of the pointed end of the almond, then squeeze the almond out of its skin into your other hand.

SUNFLOWER ALMOND MILK (*Makes 4 cups*)

¼ c. sunflower seeds	3 c. water
¼ c. almonds	1 tsp. honey

Grind the nuts and seeds in a dry blender. Add the honey and water. Blend again.

SESAME MILK (*Makes 1 cup*)

2 Tbl. sesame seeds or 1½ Tbl. 1 c. water
   tahini   ¼ tsp. honey

Grind the sesame seeds. Then, in a blender, blend the ground seeds, water and honey. (If necessary, grind the seeds in a nut-seed grinder, then transfer to blender.)

RECIPES FOR "BREAKFAST IN A GLASS"

SUNFLOWER BREAKFAST

2 tsp. ground of each:

sunflower seeds
almonds

Blend well with:

1 c. water and ¼c. tofu

Optional:

Add 1 tsp. carob powder, 1 tsp. vanilla and 1 tsp. honey.

CHERRY BREAKFAST

1 tsp. ground of each:
sunflower seeds   flax seeds
sesame seeds   almonds
pumpkin seeds   chia seeds

Blend well with:

¼ c. tofu   1½ c. water
   1 tsp. black cherry concentrate

Optional:

Add ½ banana

EGG NOG (*Serves 1*)

For a dairy-free egg nog, blend a raw organic egg and a pinch of nutmeg in the basic almond milk.

See recipes for Protein Punch and Pineapple Green Drink for other "Breakfasts in a Glass."

SMOOTHIES AND SHAKES

The combinations for smoothies are unlimited. Refer to *Blending Magic* by Dr. Bernard Jensen, for a wealth of recipes. Here are a few good combinations to blend in your blender:

½ banana + ½ c. pineapple juice   ½ banana + ½ c. apple juice

½ banana + ½ c. coconut juice
    and ¼ c. pineapple juice

Use any fruits, nuts and seeds, nut milks or fruit juices in any combination. Sliced fresh fruit, such as mango or papaya, blended with water is delicious by itself as a smoothie, or put the mixture in a popsickle mold and freeze it.

BANANA SHAKE

1 ripe, peeled banana   ¼ tsp. honey
1 c. almond milk (see "Nut Milk"),
    or 1 c. water + 1 Tbl. tahini

Blend well in a blender.

Variations:

For a carob shake, add to the banana shake 1 Tbl. unsweetened carob powder and more honey to taste.

For a mocha shake, add to the carob shake 1 tsp. cafix. Whey powder can also be added to the carob or mocha shake.

BANAN-ALMOND FIG SHAKE

In a blender, blend till creamy:

½ c. almond milk (See p. 143)   1 tsp. rice polishings
1 ripe peeled banana
2 black mission figs, soaked
   overnight, then chopped

TOFU MALT

Blend in a blender:

¼ c. ground almonds   1 Tbl. honey
¼ c. water   ¼ c. tofu
1 Tbl. unsweetened carob powder

FENUGREEK FLUFF

¼ c. fenugreek seeds
2 c. water and/or pineapple juice

Soak the seeds in the liquid all day. That night, blend the seeds and liquid together. Let the mixture sit overnight. If your blender is strong enough, blend the mixture again the next morning. If not, refrigerate as is. This is your stock. It should be quite thick and smooth. Do not be concerned if the stock is not very smooth, as you will be blending it again. The stock will keep, refrigerated for several days in a closed glass or porcelain container.

To ¼ c. stock, add and blend well in a blender 1 c. water or juice, and any of the following for flavor and nutritional variety:

   unsweetened carob powder
   pure vanilla or almond extract
   fresh fruit: raspberries, peaches, papaya, banana, blueberries, etc.

VEGGIE COCKTAILS

Vegetables can be juiced, or can be blended in a liquid (especially in the case of leafy greens).

Vegetables to juice:

carrots	celery	beets
cabbage	potatoes	turnips
parsnips	cucumbers	tomatoes

These vegetables are better juiced for a veggie cocktail. Blending them will make a raw soup.

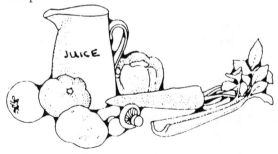

Leafy greens to juice, or blend in blender:

comfrey	parsley	basil
kale	spinach	wheatgrass
turnip greens	Swiss chard	watercress
arugula	sorrel	dill
dandelion greens	Romaine lettuce	

Leafy greens can be juiced, or can be blended very well in a liquid such as pineapple juice or a special herb tea, such as peach leaf, raspberry leaf or oatstraw.

Optional vegetable cocktail additions:

freshly squeezed lemon or lime juice
minced garlic or onion
kelp or salt-free vegetable powder

RECIPES FOR VEGGIE COCKTAILS

Suggested combinations to juice:

- carrot, celery, beet
- carrot, celery, beet, parsley
- fresh ginger, carrot
- cabbage, celery, parsley
- potato, beet
- carrot, apple

Please note: When using beet, do not use a beet larger than the size of a golf ball per person. It is heavily cleansing, and too much beet juice can cause unpleasant detoxification reactions. (Beets can also turn your eliminations red.) This is also true of certain bitter greens, such as watercress. Use only a small handful at a time. Mother Nature protects us by making such foods too bitter to overeat. Keep that in mind when juicing.

MIXED VEGETABLE JUICE (*Makes 2 c.*)

½ c. carrot juice
2 tsp. chopped parsley
1 tsp. lemon juice
powdered kelp or dulse to taste

½ c. celery juice
1 c. tomato juice
⅛ tsp. basil

Mix well.

BRILLIANT MARY (*Serves 1*)

8 oz. tomato juice
   pinch of cayenne pepper

1 clove finely minced garlic
   juice of ½ lemon

Optional:

Add 1 oz. celery juice, 1 tsp. soy sauce, or ½ tsp. horseradish.

PINEAPPLE COCKTAILS

PROTEIN PUNCH (*Makes 1¾ c.*)

Soak 1 tsp. of the following overnight in pineapple juice:

almonds
chia seeds
flax seeds

sunflower seeds
pumpkin seeds
sesame seeds

In the morning, blend well, in a blender, with 1½ c. of any of the
following liquids:

water, or water and pineapple juice
pineapple juice
chamomile, oatstraw or raspberry leaf tea

PINEAPPLE GREEN DRINK

To 1 c. pineapple juice (or ½ cup each of pineapple juice and water, if you prefer it a little less sweet) add and blend well, in a blender, the following:

1–2 sprigs watercress	1 large leaf Romaine lettuce
1 handful parsley	1 large spinach leaf

Add more liquid, if necessary. If available, add 2 small leaves fresh basil or mint.

Optional:

Add 1 raw organic egg, and/or some nuts and seeds, such as the "Protein Punch" mixture.

PINEAPPLE DRINK VARIATIONS

(Also see "Smoothies")

In a blender, blend 1 cup pineapple juice with any of the following:

1 organic egg and/or ½–1 banana	½ c. fresh carrot juice and 1 tsp. lemon juice
1 c. apple juice and 1 banana	ground nuts and seeds
1 c. coconut water and 1 c. papaya juice	fresh or frozen strawberries

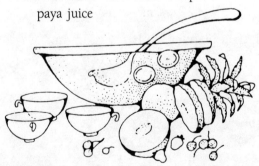

PINEAMILE PUNCH

Thanks to Eva Graf for this recipe.

1 tsp. chamomile flowers	1 tsp. honey, or more to taste
1 c. water, brought to the boil	1 c. pineapple juice

Pour the water over the chamomile flowers. Steep 15 minutes, then strain. Add honey. Let cool, then mix with pineapple juice. This is delicious hot or cold.

Punch alternatives and variations:

Use papaya juice instead of pineapple juice.
Add spearmint or peppermint leaves when steeping the tea.
Add one whole clove and/or a pinch of cinnamon when steeping.

OTHER JUICED FRUITS

HOT MULLED JUICE

To 1 quart apple cider or pineapple juice add:

2 cinnamon sticks	pinch allspice
4–5 cloves	Opt: lemon juice to taste.
pinch ground nutmeg	

Bring the juice and spices close to the boil, then turn the heat down to the lowest possible setting. Use a flame tamer, if possible. Cover the pot. Let simmer 20 minutes.

CRANBERRY JUICE

Thanks to Eva Graf for this recipe.

1 lb. cranberries	1 tsp. freshly squeezed lemon juice
2 qts. water	honey to taste

Put the cranberries and water in a large soup pot (2–3 qt. capacity). Place on a medium hot burner.

As soon as bubbles begin to form, cover the pot and take off the stove. Do not allow to boil. (Boiling cranberries releases oxalic acid which can be detrimental in excess.)

Let the cranberries sit, covered, for 25 minutes.

Separate most of the juice from the berries and put the juice aside.

Blend the berries and a little juice. Strain the mixture, throwing away the pulp.

Combine the strained mixture and the juice, and add honey to taste.

SPECIAL SOFT DRINKS

FRUIT FIZZ

Mix chilled mineral water or salt-free seltzer water with an equal amount of fruit juice, such as apple, pineapple, grape or cranberry. Or, stir 1 tsp. of pure fruit concentrate, such as black cherry concentrate, into 1 cup of the fizzy water.

HERBAL GINGER ALE

¼ tsp. powdered ginger   1 small bottle chilled mineral
¼ c. hot water   water
¼ tsp. (more or less) honey

Steep the ginger in the hot water for 10 minutes. Add the honey. Let cool, then add the mineral water.

GRAIN WATER RECIPES

Any other grain, such as rice, rye or millet can also be used by themselves or in combination.

BARLEY WATER

1 Tbl. uncooked barley   2 c. water
Raw honey, barley malt or molasses to taste after blending, if desired.

Bring the water close to the boil, turn the heat down to the lowest possible setting, cover the pot and let simmer ½ hour. Then, in a blender, blend the grain in the water until smooth and, if you prefer, strain the remaining grain pieces out.

For a nutty taste, lightly roast the grain in a dry pan before cooking it.

Grain Water Variation:

For a variety in nourishment, blend into the grain water raw greens or vegetables. If necessary, strain. For example, in a blender, blend raw kale or parsley and barley water.

Rejuvelac (Fermented Grain Water)

For the value of "rejuvelac," see p. 139.

1 c. soft pastry wheat berries,   3 c. water
   rye berries or barley

Wash the grain by rinsing it well. Allow dead seeds to float to the top, and remove them. Put the grain in a large bowl. Cover with the 3 c. water. Allow enough room at the top of the bowl for the grain to expand and the water level to rise about 4 inches. Put a clean cloth over the bowl and let it sit for 24 to 48 hours. (If you like a tangy taste, 48 hours is better.)

After the allowed soaking time, drain the fermented grain water into a pitcher, keeping the grain in the first bowl. Add 2 more cups of water to the grain and let sit another 24 hours.

After the second 24 hours, drain the fermented water into the first batch of fermented grain water, combining them.

If you like, soak the berries a third time and combine with the other batch.

If the berries are not too glutenous, you can grind them for cereal or for raw bread.

HERB TEAS

There is as much variety in herb teas as there is in plants and spices. Experiment to find the one you most enjoy.

PREPARING HERB TEAS

For leaves and flowers:

Put the herb in a tea pot or in a cup. In a saucepan or tea kettle, bring the water just to the boil, then pour over the herb.

Cover the pot or cup and let the herb steep 10–20 minutes.

For roots and pits:

Bring the water and the herb just to the boil, then turn the heat down to the lowest possible heat and let simmer 20 minutes.

Use approximately 1 tsp. dried herb per cup of water.
Pour the herb tea into a cup through a non-aluminum strainer.
Add honey, if you like.

Note that herb teas can also be used as a base for a blender drink or for cooking grains as a way of providing additional nutritional support and boosting flavor.

HERB TEA RECIPES

MINT REFRESHER

To 8 oz. peppermint or spearmint tea, add 1 tsp. honey and 1 tsp. lemon juice.

For a summer refresher, make the tea extra strong, add more honey, let cool, then add ice cubes.

SPECIAL CALCIUM TEA

1 tsp. chamomile flowers	1 tsp. alfalfa
1 tsp. oatstraw	2 c. water
1 tsp. dried comfrey	

Put the herbs in a pot. Bring the water just to the boil. Pour the water over the herbs, cover the pot, and let steep 20 minutes.

TUMMY SOOTHER

Mix together the following:

1 tsp. dried peppermint leaves	1 tsp. dried ground fennel
1 tsp. dried chamomile flowers	

Steep in 2 c. water.
Add ½ tsp. honey.
Let cool, then add ¼ c. papaya juice, or 1 Tbl. fresh papaya blended in water.

This tea has a light licorice taste.

SPECIAL LIQUID TREATS

HONIGAR

½ tsp. apple cider vinegar
½ tsp. honey
1 c. water

Optional: add a pinch of cayenne pepper

For a great pick-me-up, mix the above well, and sip with or between meals. (You may need to warm the water slightly in order to dissolve the honey.)

Note: A stock of apple cider vinegar and honey mixture can be made up and kept in the refrigerator. Use 1 tsp. stock per glass of water.

POTATO PEELING BROTH

1 organic potato
1 large carrot
2 celery stalks

1 handful parsley
3 c. water

Scrub and peel the potato, cutting the peeling ¼ inch thick. Save the potato for another recipe. Chop the carrot and celery.

On the lowest possible heat, simmer the potato peels, parsley, chopped carrot and celery for 20 minutes. Strain the vegetables out and drink the liquid broth or use as a base for any recipe that needs a stock.

Soups

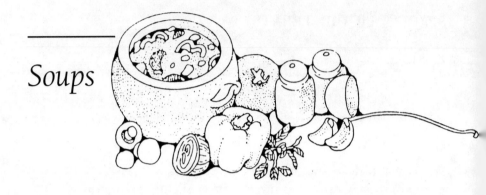

Soups are a wonderful pleasure food. They can be comforting and nourishing on a rainy or cold winter day, or lightly filling when it is too hot to eat. Soup can be a great appetizer, or a hearty meal in itself.

Soups can also provide creative ways to use left-overs and to add a lot of variety to your diet.

Soups are also perfect for convalescing and, depending on how they are prepared and which ingredients are used, can provide crucial nourishment for special health problems.

Following are suggested ingredients for soups, suggested techniques for soup preparation, and actual soup recipes.

SUGGESTED SOUP INGREDIENTS

Liquid stocks:

water
water from steaming vegetables
herb tea
vegetable juices: warm or cold, fresh or pure bottled
fruit juices: fresh or pure unsweetened bottled
nut or grain milks

vegetable bouillon (water + a bouillon cube or powder)
miso bouillon (see "Miso Soup" recipe)

Soup bases:

Vegetables: fresh, raw vegetables, left-over salad. Lightly cooked
  vegetables and left-over cooked vegetables. This also includes
  leafy greens.
Fruits: fresh, or soaked dried
Whole grains: ground or whole, freshly cooked or left over
Beans: freshly cooked or left over
Chicken: freshly cooked or left over
Fish: raw or freshly cooked
Whole grain noodles: freshly cooked or left over
Nuts and/or seeds: whole or ground
Sprouts

Flavorings:

spices, garlic, leeks, scallions, onions
fresh ginger
olive, sunflower or sesame oil
tahini or almond butter
honey, molasses, maple syrup, barley malt or rice bran syrup
apple cider vinegar
soy sauce, miso, kelp or dulse
lemon or lime juice

Thickeners:

rolled oats
ground nuts or seeds
ground raw or cooked grain
whole grain flour
kuzu or agar agar

SOUP PREPARATION

Soup Cooked in a Pot

Prepare as follows:
  (a) Optional: Slightly heat in a soup pot a small amount of oil or water. Add onions or garlic and sauté.
  (b) Add any of the following bases:
      cooked grain
      cooked pasta
      cooked fish or chicken
      cooked beans
      nuts or seeds: ground or whole
      lightly steamed vegetables
      raw, sliced or chopped vegetables
(If you are going to blend the soup, the vegetables do not have to be chopped very small.)

  (c) Add water or stock, covering the soup base. If you want a more liquid soup, add extra stock.
  (d) Bring the water or stock close to the boil. Shut the heat off, cover the pot and let the ingredients sit till warm or slightly soft. Root vegetables such as potatoes, turnips, etc. take longer. Don't overcook.
  (e) Add spices to taste.

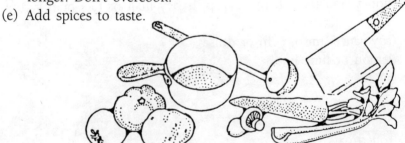

BLENDED SOUPS

There are many kinds of blended soups. Here are a few varieties with which to experiment:

RAW VEGETABLE #1:

(a) Slightly chop the raw vegetables.
(b) Put the vegetables in the blender.
(c) Add hot or cold stock, as desired, and blend.

For example, see "Quick Gaspacho for One," p. 172 and "Quick Borscht," p. 171.

Optional:

Put some of the chopped vegetables aside and add them after blending the other vegetables if you want a crunchy texture.

If you want a creamy texture, add any of the thickeners listed on page 159, and blend again.

RAW VEGETABLE #2:

(a) Juice some vegetables.
(b) Add chopped vegetables and spices.
(c) Eat cold, or warm the soup slightly over a low heat.
(d) Blend, or eat as is.

QUICK CREAMY ROOT VEGETABLE SOUP

(a) Put your choice of vegetables in a pot. See suggested combinations below.

(b) Add enough water, vegetable juice or stock to cover the vegetables.

(c) Bring the water close to the boil, shut the heat off, cover the pot and let the vegetables cook in their own steam.

(d) When the vegetables are slightly soft, put the entire pot contents (liquid plus vegetables) in the blender, and blend.

(e) Add more liquid and/or spices if necessary.

Note: If you want a crunchier texture, don't blend all the vegetables. Put some aside, and add them after blending.

Suggested Combinations for Quick-Cooked Blended Vegetable Soups:

potato + garlic and/or watercress
potato + leek
potato + celery and watercress
potato + zucchini and leek
carrot + leek and dill
carrot + onion and coriander
parsnip + scallion and mushroom
parsnip + butter and/or soy sauce
turnip + butter and/or soy sauce
squash + butter and/or soy sauce
red potato + leek and coriander
sweet potato + butter and cinnamon

Notes: Use only small amounts of watercress, as if is heavily cleansing, though nutritionally a wonderful food.

Potato soups are good hot or cold. If you like, add plain yogurt, chopped chives, and/or cucumber. Blend again and refrigerate.

Substitute "better butter" (p. 36) for butter.

Quick Creamy Grain or Bean Soup

The technique described on the previous page can be used to prepare a creamy grain or bean soup, but the grains or beans will have to be cooked more than the vegetables. For example, for quick, creamy split pea or lentil soup, low-simmer ⅓ c. split peas or lentils and two cups water for 40 minutes. Then blend the beans and the water. Refer to the grain and bean cooking charts, pp. 224 and 225 for cooking times.

Three good combinations for creamy grain or bean soups are the following:

Cooked barley + water + parsley
Cooked aduki beans or black beans + water + small amount chopped celery leaves + small amount grated lemon peel

Blended Left Overs:

(a) Put left-over salad, steamed vegetables, cooked grains or beans in the blender.
(b) And hot or cold water, soy or nut milk, or stock.
(c) Blend and add spices to taste.

For example: Zucchini-tomato sauté is delicious blended with fresh or pure bottled tomato or vegetable juice. It makes a quick gaspacho soup.

Another example: Blend cooked pumpkin, squash, carrots or sweet potato with your favorite soy milk or nut milk and/or water. For extra flavor, add scallions sautéed in a little butter. Herbs can also be added to taste, such as dill added to the carrot soup.

CREATE-A-SOUP

Another excellent technique for preparing soups is by using your steamer to create your own soup recipe. Simply steam some ingredients over a broth for about 10 minutes. Then add the steamed ingredients to the broth.

The broth can be water or juice, such as tomato or beet juice. You can also create a miso broth by adding miso paste. Add it after cooking; otherwise, you will destroy the beneficial properties in the miso and alter the flavor.

Herbs or spices, such as garlic or ginger can be added to the broth before the steaming begins. As the broth simmers under the steamer, the herbs will add flavor to the broth and to the ingredients being steamed.

While the broth is simmering, other foods can be cooked in the broth underneath the steamer, such as fish or noodles. This works well if you are preparing a quick soup for one person, since you won't need a large amount of fish or noodles. Larger amounts won't fit underneath the average steamer.

Ingredients to put in the steamer are any of the following: vegetables, fish, cooked chicken, cooked grain or cooked beans.

It takes only about eight to 10 minutes to cook the vegetables, fish or noodles, or to warm the cooked chicken, grain or beans.

After the ingredients in the steamer are cooked or warmed, empty them into the broth. If you prefer a "meal" to a soup, you can separate the ingredients out from the broth.

On the following page is a chart showing six different types of soups which you can create with this technique. Use these as examples to stimulate your own creativity. The advantage in this technique is that it is fast, and you can use foods on hand.

CREATE - A - SOUP

These delicious, hearty soups take minutes to prepare: Use the same format to create your own recipes

SOUP	BROTH LIQUID	BROTH INGREDIENTS	INGREDIENTS TO STEAM	ADDITIONAL INGREDIENTS
MISO	1 c. water		½ c. diced tofu ⅓ c. sliced Jerusalem artichoke 1 small carrot, sliced	2 tsp. miso stirred with the broth until dissolved. 1 Tbl. chopped scallions.
VEGETABLE	¼ c. water ¾ c. tomato juice	1 tsp. thyme	1 small carrot, sliced 1 small potato, diced 1 ripe tomato, chopped ¼ zucchini, sliced	1 Tbl. chopped parsley Cayenne pepper to taste
CHICKEN NOODLE	2 c. water	1 large clove garlic, minced 1 oz. whole grain fettucini noodles	6 okra, sliced, after removing the ends (or, use 1 stalk celery, chopped) 1 c. chopped, cooked chicken (without skin) 2 Tbl. sliced mushrooms	1 Tbl. chopped parsley ½ tsp. tarragon
TOMATO FISH	2 c. water	1 large clove garlic, minced 1 tsp. thyme	1 tomato, chopped ¾ c. diced, raw fish (such as cod or haddock)	1 Tbl. chopped parsley Cayenne pepper to taste
MISO FISH	2 c. water	1 large clove garlic, minced 2 tsp. minced ginger	1 small carrot, sliced ¾ c. diced, raw fish 3 1" pieces wakame seaweed	2 tsp. miso, stirred into the broth until dissolved
BEET	½ c. water ½ c. beet juice	1 tsp. caraway seeds	¼ c. sliced leeks ½ c. chopped cabbage	Optional, 1 Tbl. kefir cheese or plain yogurt

Directions:

Put the broth liquids in a medium-sized pot (8½" x 7" is perfect). Bring the liquid close to a boil. Add the "broth ingredients."
Turn the heat down to a low simmer.
Put a vegetable steamer in the pot. Put the "ingredients to steam" in the steamer.
Cover the pot. Simmer on a low heat for 8 minutes, or until the vegetables are slightly soft, and the chicken is warm, or the fish is cooked.
Turn the heat off. Empty the steamed ingredients into the broth. Add the "additional ingredients." Serves 1.

SOUP RECIPES

VEGETABLE SOUP (*Serves 4*)

2 tsp. olive oil	1 leaf cabbage, torn into pieces
1 large onion, chopped	2 stalks celery, chopped
1–2 cloves garlic, minced	1 potato, diced
4 c. water	½ turnip, diced
1 vegetable cube or 1 tsp. powder	2 tomatoes, diced
2 carrots, chopped	1 small bay leaf
	⅛ tsp. thyme

Warm the olive oil on a low heat in a large pot. Add the onions and garlic and sauté till soft. Add the water. Stir the vegetable cube or powder till dissolved. Add the remaining ingredients.

Bring the water close to the boil. Turn the heat off, cover the pot and let the vegetables sit till slightly soft, but still crunchy.

Optional:

Add cayenne pepper or miso paste to taste, after cooking.

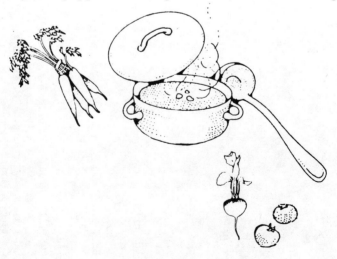

QUICK CHICKEN OR FISH NOODLE SOUP (*Makes about 2½ c.*)

1 clove garlic, minced
4 large mushrooms, chopped
2 tsp. olive oil
2 c. water
1 oz. whole grain noodles
¼ tsp. thyme
½ c. sliced okra (optional)

1 c. diced cooked chicken or diced raw fish (such as cod or haddock)
1 Tbl. chopped parsley
½ large tomato, chopped
pinch cayenne pepper

Warm the olive oil on a low heat in a soup pan. Add the garlic and mushrooms. Sauté till they are soft. Add the water, noodles and thyme.

Low simmer 5 minutes. Add the remaining ingredients, except the cayenne, and low simmer another 3 minutes. Add the cayenne.

ONION SOUP (*Serves 4*)

olive oil
6 medium white onions, sliced thin
pinch cumin
6 c. water

1 minced clove garlic
½ tsp. mustard
1 vegetable cube or 1 tsp. powder

Cover the bottom of the pot with a thin layer of olive oil. Heat the oil slightly, then add the onions, garlic, and mustard. Sauté on a low heat till the onions are lightly brown. Add a pinch of cumin, the water and the vegetable cube.

Bring the water just to the boil, cover the pot, then turn the heat down to a low simmer for about 45 minutes.

Before serving, add 2 tsp. soy sauce and more cumin and cayenne pepper to taste.

MISO SOUP (*Serves 4*)

4 c. water	4 scallions, chopped
A few pieces of seaweed (wakame or dulse)	3 carrots, sliced or diced
	4 Tbl. miso paste

Optional:

½ cube of tofu, broken into small chunks
1 Jerusalem artichoke (sunchoke), sliced
minced garlic, and/or ginger to taste

Put the seaweed, scallions, carrots and water into the pot. Add the minced garlic and/or ginger and the sunchokes.

Bring the water close to the boiling point.

Add the tofu, cover the pot, turn the heat off, and let the vegetables sit, covered, till slightly soft (8 to 10 minutes).

Put the miso paste in a cup or small bowl. Ladle a small amount of the soup broth into the bowl and stir till the miso is dissolved. Empty the miso broth into the soup and stir. Do not let miso boil, as the high heat will stop the beneficial enzyme activity, and distorts the flavor.

Note: Miso broth makes a great, hearty soup base, especially for a winter soup.

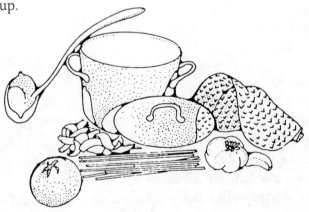

LENTIL-TOMATO SOUP *(Serves 4)*

2 Tbl. olive oil
1 onion, chopped
2 cloves garlic, minced
5 c. water or stock
⅔ c. lentils
4 small carrots, sliced

2 stalks celery, chopped
3 Tbl. pure tomato paste
¼ tsp. thyme
pinch tarragon
chopped parsley for garnish

Warm the olive oil in a large soup pot. Sauté the onion and garlic in the olive oil. Add the water, lentils, thyme and tarragon. Bring the water to a boil, lower the heat and cook, covered, till the lentils are soft (25 to 30 minutes.) Add the carrots, celery and tomato paste. Cook till carrots are soft (about 10 minutes) and flavors are blended.

LEMON-EGG SOUP *(Serves 2–3)*

(This is a great way to use leftover rice)

3 c. water
3 bouillon cubes
4 large cloves garlic
1 bay leaf

1 cup cooked brown rice
1 Tbl. butter
2 eggs
juice of one lemon

Bring the water to a boil in a soup pot. Add the bouillon cubes, the bay leaf and the garlic. Simmer at the lowest possible temperature for 30–40 minutes, allowing the garlic flavor to permeate the water.

Remove and discard the bay leaf and garlic.

A few minutes before the above process is completed, heat the rice in a separate pan in the butter, and beat the eggs with the lemon juice.

About 5–10 minutes before serving the soup, add some of the hot broth mixture to the beaten egg/lemon mixture. Stir vigorously, then return the broth/lemon/egg mixture to the soup pot.

Continue to stir the soup broth and to heat it for a few minutes on a low temperature, until the egg mixture is smoothly blended into the broth.

Add the cooked rice and serve at once.

Garnish each bowl of soup with a paper thin slice of lemon, and, if you like, a sprig of parsley or watercress.

BLENDED SOUP RECIPES

RAW SPINACH SOUP (*Makes 3 cups*)

Blend well in the blender:

¼ c. almonds
1 c. tomato juice
1 c. water
2 c. raw spinach
1 small clove garlic, minced
1 Tbl. chopped scallion (1 thin scallion)

½ c. packed celery leaves
⅜ tsp. ground cumin or ⅛ tsp. ground nutmeg
⅛ tsp. kelp, dulse powder or vegetable salt

After blending the above mixture, gradually add and blend in a second cup of water, blending to the consistency you like.

Note that the taste will be completely different if you use nutmeg in place of cumin. If you aren't sure which to use, empty small amounts of the mixture into two cups. Then add a pinch of nutmeg to one cup, and two pinches of cumin to the other. They are both good!

RAW BORSCHT (*Makes 4 cups*)

¾ c. fresh or pure bottled beet
   juice
1½ tsp. dried dill, or caraway
   seeds
½ tsp. soy sauce

1 Tbl. lemon juice
1 clove garlic, minced
1¼ c. water
⅓ c. tomato juice

In a blender, blend the above, then add:
1½ c. chopped cucumber.

Blend slightly until the cucumber is well mixed, but not liquified.
   Garnish with sliced cucumbers and/or dill.
   For a quick cold borscht for one person, blend 1 small beet, 1
c. water, chopped cucumber (3 times more cucumber than beet),
and lemon juice, dill or caraway to taste.
   For a delicious hot borscht for one which does not require a
blender, see Create-A-Soup p. 165.
   Please note: For some people, beet juice will stain their eliminations red. Beets, though a great liver support, are heavily cleansing,
so do not use more than a beet the size of a golf ball per person,
or ⅓ c. juice per person.

SWEET POTATO OR SQUASH SOUP (*Makes 6 cups*)

In a blender, blend well:

4 c. cooked sweet potato or winter squash, such as pumpkin,
   acorn or butternut
2½ c. water

2 Tbl. melted butter
⅓ c. chopped scallion, lightly
   sauteed in butter

GAZPACHO (*Serves 4*)

½ c. water
2 c. tomato juice
2 tsp. lemon juice
3 Tbl. chopped scallions (about 1 scallion)
1 clove garlic, minced
2 Tbl. chopped green pepper

1 tsp. basil
½ tsp. chervil
2 pinches cayenne pepper
½ tsp. kelp, optional
1 Tbl. chopped parsley
1 small cube of a beet, optional

Blend the above thoroughly in the blender; then stir in without blending:

1 c. chopped tomatoes
½ c. chopped celery
½ c. chopped zucchini

2 c. peeled and chopped cucumber

Garnish with parsley and a slice of lemon.

QUICK GAZPACHO FOR ONE

Blend any fresh vegetables (or cooked left overs) in one cup fresh or bottled tomato juice.

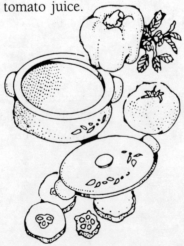

POTATO LEEK SOUP (*Serves 4*)

3 Tbl. butter

3 large potatoes, sliced fine

2 medium sized leeks, sliced

1½ c. water

½ tsp. mustard

1 c. plain yogurt

parsley to garnish

Melt the butter on a low heat in a large saucepan. Add the potatoes, leeks, mustard and water. Bring the water close to the boiling point. Shut the heat off and let sit, covered, till the potatoes and leeks are slightly soft.

Blend the entire pot contents in the blender, adding more water if you like. Add the yogurt and blend again. If necessary, rewarm, but be careful not to boil, as it spoils the yogurt and gives it a metallic taste.

QUICK POTATO SOUP FOR ONE

1½ c. water

½ large potato, chopped in chunks

Put the potato and the water in a soup pot. Bring the water close to the boil. Cover the pot, shut off the heat and let the potato cook in its own steam till slightly soft.

Put the potato and water in the blender and blend well.

If you like, add any of the following while blending:

butter   soy sauce   chives   cucumber

minced garlic   watercress   parsley

Use this same recipe for any root vegetable or any combination of vegetables: parsnips, turnips, daikon radish, carrots, etc.

Salads

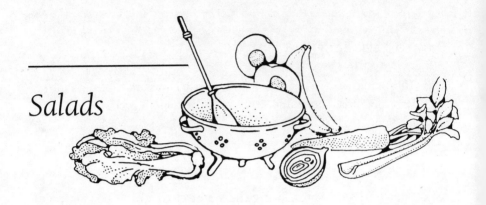

Salads can be the most important part of your meal since they can provide you with a variety of nutrients, fiber and vitality. And, they can give you the most pleasure—in their beauty, their delicious taste, and in the opportunity for you to be creative.

Salads can be created from any type of food in any combination. Experiment with the varieties of colors, flavors, textures and shapes. This is Mother Nature's way of letting us know we are getting a good variety of nutrients, without needing to know the chemical breakdown of foods.

Experiment to your heart's delight.

SUGGESTED SALAD INGREDIENTS

Cooked grains
Cooked pasta
Cooked chicken
Cooked or raw fish
Cooked beans
Tofu
Sprouts
Vegetables: chopped, sliced, grated, diced, or eaten finger-sized.

Leafy greens such as Romaine lettuce, parsley, watercress, raw
    spinach, etc.
Fruits: fresh, or dried and rehydrated (soaked).
Nuts and seeds: whole, ground, soaked or chopped.
Fresh herbs or flowers

VEGETABLE & FRUIT SALAD RECIPES

Please note: For pasta salads, grain salads, bean salads and chicken
salads, refer to the individual sections.

If you are not sure of the identification of certain vegetables,
such as Jerusalem artichoke (or sunchoke), see the drawings on
pages 40–41.

QUICK SALADS

SALAD ON THE GO

Washing and chopping ahead of time is generally not recommended,
since it results in loss of nutrients and vitality. Occasionally, however, you could pre-cut and refrigerate some leafy greens and raw
vegetables. Eat them as a quick snack with a dip. Or, combine them
in a last-minute salad and mix with a pre-made dressing.

You could also pre-cook beans, grains and chicken. Keep them
in separate containers. Combine them as you like with the vegetables
and/or cooked noodles. Again, top with a pre-made dip or dressing,
such as the tofu dip, p. 190, mustard dressing, p. 249, or Ruth
Duffy's Tarragon Dressing, p. 187.

CARROT SALAD

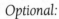

4 c. grated carrots (about 3 medium carrots)
½ c. chopped walnuts
½ c. soaked currants or raisins

1 c. diced apples and/or
pineapple
2 Tbl. shredded coconut

Optional:

½ c. sunflower seeds

Mix and decorate with sprigs of parsley. Top with honey dressing, p. 188.

AVOCADO-WATERCRESS SALAD

Combine sliced avocado and watercress leaves. (Save the hard watercress stems for your green drink.)
   Squeeze lemon juice over the avocado and watercress, then sprinkle soy sauce on top.

Optional additions:

sesame seeds   tofu chunks   raw peas
raw zucchini   raw string beans   sprouts
slices of raw Jerusalem artichoke (sunchoke)

Note: For a longer (but delicious!) version of the avocado watercress
salad, and to serve 4 people, use ¾ bunch of watercress leaves and
1 ripe avocado. Top with the following dressing:

4 Tbl. extra virgin olive oil
2 cloves garlic, minced
4 tsp. sesame seeds

2 Tbl. soy sauce
2½ Tbl. lemon juice

Sauté the garlic in the oil on a low heat for approximately 2 minutes,
stirring constantly. Add the sesame seeds. Continue to sauté for 1

minute longer, taking care that the seeds don't burn. Remove from heat. Add the soy sauce and lemon juice. Make a bed of watercress on 4 individual salad plates. Top with sliced avocado, then the dressing.

TOMATO-BASIL SALAD

Slice a fresh, ripe tomato. Top with fresh basil and a good quality olive oil.

BLENDED SALAD

In a blender, blend well in the order listed:

juice from ½ lemon	½ green pepper
1 Tbl. sesame or sunflower oil	2–3 leaves Romaine lettuce
1 wedge of a ripe tomato	1–2 stalks celery
1 small cucumber, sliced and peeled	

Optional:

Add spices of your choice, such as minced garlic or a pinch of cayenne pepper.

This salad will have a mushy texture. It is an excellent salad for those who have extreme dental or digestive difficulty.

WATERCRESS–ENDIVE SALAD

1 c. sliced endive

1 c. watercress sprigs (Save the hard stems for your green drink.)

12 pecans, chopped

Mix and top with Ruth Duffy's Tarragon Dressing, p. 187. This salad is delicious with Italian Tofu and Pasta, p. 240.

AVOCADO-SUNCHOKE SALAD

3 Jerusalem artichokes, sliced thin

1 ripe avocado, pitted, peeled and diced

½ c. mung bean sprouts

¼ c. alfalfa sprouts

1 c. shredded Romaine lettuce

Mix all ingredients well, then sprinkle with lemon juice to taste.

RAW VEGETABLE SNACKS

Raw vegetables are wonderful snacks—plain, or with dips or sauces.
Use any of the following:

cherry tomatoes

carrot slices

broccoli flowers

turnip slices

sweet potato slices

sliced bell peppers

cauliflowerettes

sliced Jerusalem artichokes
   (sunchokes)

raw peas

celery slices

green string beans

radish roses

yellow snap beans

mushrooms

cucumber slices

Arrange the vegetables in a beautiful manner in baskets or on a
plate. Put the vegetables on a bed of Romaine and/or purple head
lettuce and decorate with slivers of purple cabbage, radish roses,
cherry tomatoes and large sprigs of parsley or watercress.
   Or, carry them in a baggie as a snack, along with a container of
nut butter or dip. (See dip recipes, pp. 190–191.)

PEA SALAD (*Serves 3*)

1 c. fresh raw peas

½ c. grated red cabbage

½ c. sliced sunchokes

2 Tbl. chopped scallions

¼ c. chopped green beans

2 Tbl. sliced radish

2 Romaine or Boston lettuce
   leaves, torn into bite sized
   pieces.

Combine, and top with tofu dressing, p. 190.

ALFALFA CROQUETTES (*Serve 2*)

Mix thoroughly:

1 c. alfalfa sprouts	2 Tbl. tahini
2 Tbl. grated red cabbage	1 tsp. lemon juice
2 Tbl. grated carrot	3 Tbl. carrot juice
4 Tbl. chopped celery	½ c. ground sunflower seeds
2 Tbl. chopped parsley	(about ⅓ c. unground seeds)
½ tsp. minced garlic	

Serving suggestions:

(1) Serve in tomato cups. Cut the tomato about ¾ of the way down, 3 ways, so that you have 6 sections connected at the bottom. After you fill them with the mixture, top with parsley sprigs and serve on a bed of lettuce.
(or)
(2) Refrigerate the mixture for 1 hour, so that it is more stiff, then form patties.

MARINATED VEGETABLES

6 cherry tomatoes, halved	1 small red onion, sliced thin
¾ lb. yellow squash, diced	¼ c. chopped parsley
¾ lb. zucchini, sliced thin	

Marinade:

¼ c. olive oil	¼ tsp. basil
¼ c. apple cider vinegar	pinch oregano
1 small clove garlic, minced	

Marinate the vegetables for 5 hours or more, stirring occasionally. Decorate with parsley.

SALT FREE SAUERKRAUT

Utensils:

3 mixing bowls
a large crock or glass pot
a plate which fits just inside the pot
a clean, white cotton cloth
a heavy weight, such as a water-filled jar

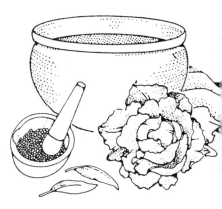

Ingredients:

1 head green cabbage and 1
   head purple cabbage, grated,
   except for the outer leaves.
   Put the outer leaves aside.
2 onions, chopped
8 cloves garlic, minced
2 carrots, grated
2 zucchini, chopped
1 head cauliflower, broken into
   flowerettes

2 stalks celery, chopped
2 beets, grated
2 Tbl. each of caraway seeds,
   dill seeds and celery seeds.
   Measure, then grind.
1 Tbl. ground kelp
2 Tbl. garlic powder

This recipe may look slightly complicated, but doing it is very simple and very rewarding. It is delicious and will keep refrigerated for weeks. Sauerkraut is an excellent source of vitamins C, B1, B2, thiamin, and riboflavin, as well as calcium, phosphorous, and lactic acid, which helps maintain a healthy bowel. The sauerkraut ferments in 8 to 10 days. It also makes great sauerkraut juice in the process.

This recipe makes several quarts. Small quantities can be prepared in the same way.

Sauerkraut preparation:

Put the grated cabbage in one mixing bowl, the prepared vegetables and onion in another bowl, and the ground spices and minced garlic in another bowl.

Put a layer of the cabbage about one inch deep in the crock or glass pot. Pack it down. Put a one inch layer of the vegetable mixture over the cabbage and pack it down. Then sprinkle with a layer of the spices. Gently mix the entire mixture and pack it down again.

Repeat the process until you are finished with the ingredients, or until you are three inches from the top of the pot. (You need space, since the water you will add will bubble and rise in the fermentation process.)

Cover the mixture with the outer leaves of the cabbage, tucking the leaves around the mixture as well as possible. Cover the leaves with the cotton cloth and tuck the cloth tightly around the mixture.

Pour water (or rejuvelac, if you want it to ferment faster. See p. 154) over the cloth and keep pouring until you see that the sauerkraut is well drenched and water is appearing above the cloth.

Put the plate on top, then the weight. Push the plate down to be sure the mixture is packed as tightly as possible.

Put a clean cloth over the pot, and put the pot in a warm place (about 70–80° F). If it has not started bubbling within 48 hours, the place is not warm enough. You can put the pot in the oven with the pilot light.

Be sure there is always enough liquid above the plate, since the liquid keeps the sauerkraut from spoiling.

When it is ready (8–10 days), skim off the scum on the surface. Gently remove the weight, plate, cloth and outer leaves plus any more scum. Drain and mix the sauerkraut, saving the juice, then refrigerate the juice and sauerkraut.

FRUIT SALAD RECIPES

AVOCADO AND PINK GRAPEFRUIT

Pit, peel and slice a ripe avocado. Cut out the sections of the grapefruit. Arrange the pieces on a bed of lettuce and top with poppy seed dressing (p.189) and a sprig of watercress.

Optional:

Add chopped pecans.

Tropical Delight

Combine in a bowl:

sliced bananas	green grapes
sliced or diced papaya	soaked currants
	or
sliced or diced mango	strawberries
diced pineapple	

Optional: Add shredded coconut.

Eat as is, or top with thick almond milk, or Quick Fruit Dressing, p. 186.

Here is an easy way to prepare a mango:

Cut just through the skin (not into the fruit) of the mango, all the way around, from end to end, on two sides. Hold the mango and peel one section, exposing the fruit. With a knife, cut the fruit off the pit. Keep peeling and cutting the fruit, holding an unpeeled section as long as possible. Eventually, there will be no more unpeeled section to hold. This method helps get more fruit off the pit with less mess.

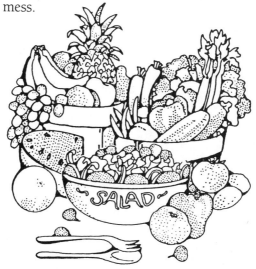

Dressings, Dips, Spreads & Sauces

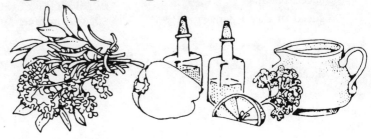

SAUCE, DIP AND DRESSING INGREDIENTS:

OILS

Cold pressed olive, sesame, sunflower, canola, walnut, flax or soy
Nut/seed butters, such as tahini, almond
Avocado

LIQUIDS

Water
Vegetable juices
Fruit juices or concentrates
Apple cider vinegar

BULK INGREDIENTS

Vegetables: raw, lightly steamed
Fruits: fresh or rehydrated dried
Cooked beans
Cooked grains
Tofu
Ground nuts and seeds

FLAVORINGS

Fresh & dried herbs and spices
Sweeteners such as honey, molasses, maple syrup, barley malt,
    fruit juice
Soy sauce
Lemon or lime juice

THICKENERS

Flour
Kuzu or arrowroot
Slippery elm powder or ground psyllium seeds

SALAD DRESSING RECIPES

Salad dressings can be made by mixing oil, vinegar or other liquids with herbs and spices. Or, in a blender, blend any fruits and
vegetables with liquid ingredients and seasonings.

Many of the dressing recipes can be used for sauces, and some of the
dip recipes can be used as dressings simply by adding more liquid for a
thinner consistency. Each recipe will note this possibility.

SUPER QUICK DRESSINGS

Lemon/Soy:

Squeeze lemon juice over steamed or raw vegetables, or avocado.
Then sprinkle soy sauce on top.

Oil/Vinegar:

Sprinkle apple cider vinegar or lemon juice over the salad, then
add the oil and spices.

Ginger/Soy:

Mix minced ginger, soy sauce and lemon juice, then put on the salad.

Quick Carrot:

Blend tofu, carrot, soy sauce and lemon juice to taste.

Blended Vegetable:

In a blender, blend any vegetables (such as tomato, green pepper, or lettuce) with apple cider vinegar, olive oil, herbs and minced garlic.

Quick Fruit Dressing or Sauce:

In a blender, blend any fruits, by themselves or together, with a small amount of water or pineapple juice. Optional: Add to taste honey, vanilla or cinnamon.
Suggested fruits: peach, pineapple, banana.

OIL AND VINEGAR

2–3 Tbl. apple cider vinegar	1 tsp. dried basil
1 pinch cayenne pepper	1 clove garlic, minced

Combine the above, then add:

¼ c. sesame oil	¼ c. olive oil

Then add any of the following:

a pinch of powdered kelp	1–2 sprigs parsley, finely chopped
⅓ tsp. soy sauce	pinch grated Parmesan cheese

Sunflower/Beet Dressing

½ c. sunflower seeds
1 c. beet juice, fresh or bottled
1½ tsp. soy sauce
1½ tsp. lemon juice

1–2 cloves garlic, minced
¼ c. each of sesame and olive oil
1½ tsp. dried dill, or to taste

Grind the sunflower seeds in a dry blender. Add the beet juice, soy sauce, lemon juice and garlic. Blend. Then, while the blender is on low, slowly add a steady stream of the ½ c. mixture of olive and sesame oils. Add minced dill.

Ruth Duffy's Tarragon Dressing

Blend well in a blender:

1 c. sesame oil
1 Tbl. tarragon
3 cloves garlic, minced

⅓ c. cider vinegar
1 tsp. celery seed
1 tsp. mustard

Tahini-Ginger Dressing or Sauce

1" piece of ginger, peeled and minced
3 garlic cloves, minced
1 c. oil (half sesame, half olive)
juice of 1 lemon

2 Tbl. tahini
2 Tbl. soy sauce

Place the garlic and the ginger in a blender. Cover with a little oil and blend to a fine paste. Add the rest of the oil, lemon juice, tahini and soy sauce. Blend again. Add more tahini if a thicker dressing is desired.

This is also a delicious sauce for grain, noodles or tofu.

WATERCRESS DRESSING

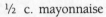

Combine in a blender and blend well:

½ c. mayonnaise

1 c. plain yogurt

1 c. chopped watercress leaves

1 Tbl. apple cider vinegar

1 Tbl. fresh lemon juice

½ tsp. soy sauce

½ tsp. minced onion

1 clove garlic, minced

CARROT-GINGER DRESSING

1 Tbl. sesame seeds

1 medium carrot, cut in 1"
  . pieces

½ c. olive oil

2 Tbl. cider vinegar

1½–2 tsp. minced fresh ginger

4 tsp. soy sauce

½–¾ c. water

Grind the sesame seeds and set aside. Chop the carrot pieces in your blender, then add sesame seeds and other ingredients and blend.

SWEET DRESSINGS

Also, see Super Quick Fruit Dressing, p. 186.

HONEY DRESSING (*Makes ⅓ cup*)

Combine and shake well before using:

½ c. sunflower or sesame oil

2 Tbl. honey

¼ tsp. lemon juice

BANANA DRESSING (*Makes 1 cup*)

Blend well in a blender:

½ c. sunflower or sesame oil	1 Tbl. lemon juice
½ c. pineapple juice	1 medium ripe banana

POPPY SEED DRESSING (*Makes 1 cup*)

Blend well in a blender:

⅓ c. honey	1 tsp. lemon juice
¼ tsp. dry mustard	¼ tsp. grated lemon peel
½ c. sesame or sunflower oil	2 tsp. onion juice
¼ c. apple cider vinegar	2 tsp. poppy seeds

PAPAYA DRESSING (*Makes 1½ cups*)

Mix well:

½ c. sunflower or sesame oil	½ c. apple cider vinegar
½ c. papaya concentrate	1 Tbl. lemon juice

Optional:

If mayonnaise is preferred, whip an egg into the mixture.

DIP RECIPES

To make these dips into dressings or sauces, simply add more liquid. For a quick dip, use nut butter, such as tahini or almond butter. Add chopped cucumber for a lighter taste.

For other dip ideas, see p. 193.

TOFU-VEGETABLE DIP, SAUCE OR DRESSING

¾ c. light olive oil
1 medium sized carrot, slightly chopped
⅔ c. chopped fresh parsley
1 tsp. white part of scallion

1 Tbl. green part of scallion
3 Tbl. lemon juice
1 clove garlic, minced
8 oz. firm tofu
1 Tbl. soy sauce

Put the olive oil and the carrot chunks in a blender and blend well. Add the parsley, scallions, lemon juice and garlic and blend well. Then add the tofu and soy sauce. Blend well again. It comes out thick, like a dip. For a sauce over steamed vegetables, or for a salad dressing, add water to thin.

Note: For a curried tofu dip, see p. 236.

GUACAMOLE (AVOCADO DIP)   *Serves 4*

2 ripe avocados, pitted and mashed
⅛ tsp. onion juice
1½ Tbl. lemon juice

12 ripe cherry tomatoes, chopped
1 large, or two small scallions, chopped

Mix all ingredients well, adding the avocado last. Serve in a bowl as a dip or spread. Or, serve in the avocado skin or in tomato cups.

SESAME TAHINI DIP, SAUCE OR DRESSING

¼ to ½ c. lemon juice
1 scallion, chopped
2 cloves garlic, minced
½ green pepper, seeded and
  chopped
¼ c. chopped parsley

½ c. water
1 c. tahini
1 pinch cayenne pepper
½ tsp. cumin
2 Tbl. soy sauce

Put the garlic, lemon juice, scallion, green pepper and parsley into the blender. Blend well until smooth.

Add the water. Then, while the blender is on low, slowly add the tahini. If it's still too thick, add more water.

Add the remaining spices and blend again.

This recipe makes a blender full of a great dip for raw vegetables. For a dressing or sauce for vegetables, grains, noodles, tofu, or beans, add more water until you reach the desired consistency.

SPRING GREEN DIP (*Makes about 1½ c.*)

2 Tbl. finely chopped red pepper and green pepper
3 Tbl. finely chopped parsley
  and scallions

⅔ c. plain yogurt
½ c. mayonnaise
  pinch cayenne

Mix the mayonnaise and the yogurt in a bowl, then add the vegetables.

Add the cayenne.

Mix well and chill.

Serve with mixed raw vegetables.

SPREADS & SAUCES RECIPES

Put sauces on cooked grains, noodles, tofu, legumes (beans), chicken or fish, loaves, steamed or raw vegetables.

THICKENERS

Two particularly good thickeners and jelling agents (which are wheat-free) are kuzu and arrowroot.

Kuzu:

There are many advantages to using kuzu as a thickener or jelling agent:

1. It has a smooth, light texture and a delicate, non-starchy flavor.
2. By adding it to sauces or frostings, you extend the amount of sauce without adding caloric ingredients such as tahini or honey, or salty ingredients such as miso.
3. When used in sweet sauces or glazes, the alkalinizing properties of the kuzu help balance the acidic properties of the sweet.

To use kuzu, mix it with cool liquid, blending or stirring till dissolved. Crush any lumps with your fingertips. If necessary, strain. Otherwise, put the mixture over a very low heat and stir constantly till thick.

The proportions of kuzu and liquid are:

Sauces: 1½ to 2¼ tsp. kuzu to 1 c.

liquid, depending on the thickness you desire

For jelling: 2 Tbl. kuzu to 1 c. liquid.

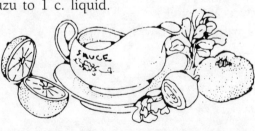

Arrowroot:

Arrowroot is less expensive than kuzu, but lacks kuzu's alkalinizing and medicinal properties and is inferior in texture. It does not make as smooth and delicate a sauce, nor as firm and cohesive a jell. However, it is perfectly adequate.

Use 1½ Tbl. arrowroot per cup of liquid to be thickened. Mix it with a small amount of the liquid first. Stir until it has dissolved and is the consistency of paste, then add it to the simmering liquid, which will then turn cloudy. Continue stirring until the liquid is clear and thick. Remove from the heat and let cool.

QUICK SAUCE OR SPREAD COMBINATIONS:

Blend well in any proportions preferred. Add water to thin, if necessary:

Mix by hand in a bowl:

- Miso paste or soy sauce + tahini and any flavorings
- Tahini + ginger
- Tahini + dulse seaweed and lemon juice
- Tahini + honey or barley malt + cinnamon (great on toast)

Blend in blender:

- Cooked millet + tahini and soy sauce
- Cooked rice + tahini and ginger
- Cooked potatoes + butter, garlic and soy sauce
- Cooked lentils + garlic, lemon juice and soy sauce
- Tofu + tahini, ginger and soy sauce

QUICK BLENDED SUPER SAUCE OR GRAVY

Put in the blender:

1½ c. water	1 Tbl. kuzu
¼ c. tahini	1 Tbl. miso
2 tsp. minced ginger	

Blend well, then cook on a low heat, stirring constantly, till thick. Refrigerate, covered.

Alternates:

Make the above gravy; however, eliminate the ginger and add any of the following:
    1 clove garlic, minced
    1½ tsp. ground cumin or 1 tsp. tarragon

BETTER BUTTER

To cut down on the amount of saturated fat and cholesterol consumed by eating butter, mix it with olive oil, a type of fat which is good for the heart. Mix softened butter with as much olive oil as possible, maintaining the butter flavor and a spreadable consistency. Store in a bowl in the refrigerator.

MISO-TAHINI SPREAD OR SAUCE

1 c. tahini	water to thin
¼–⅓ c. miso paste	

Add the miso to the tahini gradually, to taste, as miso is very salty. Add water, stirring very well, to thin. (A small amount of water, such as 2 Tbl., will still give you a spread, yet will soften the flavor and extend the amount.) Refrigerate, covered.

Use any of the following optional flavor changers:

1–2 tsp. honey
    grated fresh ginger
  1 Tbl. minced onion or garlic
    grated orange or lemon peel
    (organic)

lemon juice
½ tsp. marjoram

As a spread, it's delicious on bread, toast or crackers with sprouts or chopped watercress leaves. Or, use it as a sauce.

TOMATO SAUCES

REAL TOMATO SAUCE (*Makes about 2½ c.*)

¼ c. olive oil
1 very large onion, diced
3–4 cloves garlic, minced
¼ c. chopped mushrooms
¼ green pepper, chopped
2 Tbl. diced parsley
1 tsp. oregano
2 tsp. basil

1 bay leaf
3½ c. skinned and chopped tomatoes. (If you cannot find large, ripe tomatoes, use ripe unpeeled cherry tomatoes, or two 12 oz. cans unadulterated canned tomatoes.)

Sauté the onion, garlic and mushrooms in the olive oil till the onions are lightly browned. Add all other ingredients. Bring close to the boil, then reduce heat to lowest possible simmer. Simmer 45 minutes. Add water if it gets too thick.

No-Tomato Tomato Sauce (*makes about 4 cups*)

For those allergic to tomatoes, here is a sauce that tastes very much like tomato sauce.

2 Tbl. olive oil	1 Tbl. chopped parsley
1½ large onion, chopped	½ green pepper, seeded and
3 cloves garlic, minced	chopped

Sauté the onion and garlic in the olive oil till the onion is transparent. Put aside ½ c. of the onion/garlic mixture, the parsley, and 1 Tbl. of the chopped green pepper.

In a blender, blend well the following:

The remaining sautéed onion/ garlic mixture	2 tsp. apple cider vinegar
The rest of the green pepper	1 Tbl. minced garlic
2 medium zucchinis, chopped	1½ Tbl. olive oil
1 small to medium beet, chopped	⅔ c. water (or more, if necessary)
2 Tbl. Italian seasoning (such as 1½ Tbl. basil, 1 tsp. oregano and 1 tsp. thyme)	

After blending, return the blended mixture, along with the ingredients you put aside (½ c. onion/garlic mixture, 1 Tbl. chopped green pepper and 1 Tbl. chopped parsley) to the pan and let gently simmer on a low heat until the flavors are well blended. You may want to add more apple cider vinegar, olive oil or water.

JAMS & RELISHES

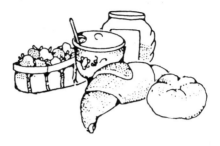

STRAWBERRY JAM

Blend well:

2 c. strawberries
½ c. honey

1 section each of an orange and
of a lemon

(You may occasionally need to turn off the blender and use a rubber spatula to push the ingredients into the center of the blender.)

Alternates:

Use dried apricots, which have been soaked for 2–3 hours. Or, use fresh peaches and eliminate the orange and lemon.

GINGERED CARROT MARMALADE

1 c. grated carrots
¾ unpeeled organic lemon,
    sliced (remove seeds)
1½ to 2 tsp. minced ginger

½ c. honey
1 Tbl. pure pectin (no sugar or
    chemicals)
2 Tbl. water

Put the carrots, lemon, ginger and water into a blender. Blend to a coarse mixture. Put the mixture in a bowl. Add the honey and pectin. Mix well. Refrigerate 3 hours, or overnight.

Note: If you don't like ginger, just eliminate it for a delicious honey marmalade.

CRANBERRY RELISH (*Makes 1½ c.*)

2 c. cranberries

½ c. honey

1 small orangic orange, with peel, cut in pieces.

Grind the cranberries in the blender, then add the orange pieces and the honey.

Chicken

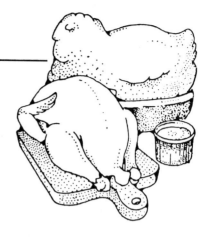

Chicken has about the same nutritional value as red meat, yet is less expensive, has less fat, and is easier to digest. However, commercial chickens are fed arsenic to stimulate appetite, and are injected with antibiotics and hormones to encourage quick, fatty growth and fast profits. Whenever possible, buy organically raised chickens. The extra cost will be balanced by increased health value.

The following chicken recipes are delicious, but sometimes it's easier and more creative to have pre-baked chicken in the refrigerator to add to salads, soups, or other recipes at the last minute.

CHICKEN RECIPES

COQ AU VIN (*Serves 4–6*)

Use a broiler or roasting chicken or 2 fryer chickens, cut into parts.

2 Tbl. olive oil	2 Tbl. chopped parsley
¾ c. diced onions	1 small bay leaf
1 clove garlic, minced	1 Tbl. chervil or marjoram
6 shallots or small white onions	¼ tsp. thyme
8 large, whole mushrooms	1½ c. dry red wine or sherry
1 medium carrot, sliced	

Preheat the oven to 325°. Wash the chicken pieces and pat them dry.

Warm the oil in a large fry pan. Brown the chicken in the oil, remove and let cool.

Remove the skin, then put the chicken in a large casserole which has a lid.

Sauté the diced onions and garlic in the juices in the fry pan.

Add the sautéed onions and garlic, the juices from the fry pan and all remaining ingredients to the chicken in the casserole. Cover and bake until done—about 1½–2 hours.

CURRIED CHICKEN (*Serves 4*)

4 boneless, skinless chicken
  breasts
2 Tbl. olive oil
1 onion, chopped (about 1½
  cups)
1 clove garlic, minced
5 mushrooms, chopped (about
  1⅓ cups)

2 Tbl. curry powder
2 Tbl. cumin
½ Tbl. turmeric
1 tsp. cardamon
2 whole cloves
1 Tbl. plain yogurt
½ cup tomato juice

Saute the onion, garlic and mushrooms in olive oil until mushrooms are light brown. Add spices, tomato juice and yogurt. Simmer 5 minutes, then add chicken. Add water till you have a sauce (about 1 cup). Simmer till chicken is done (about 35 minutes).

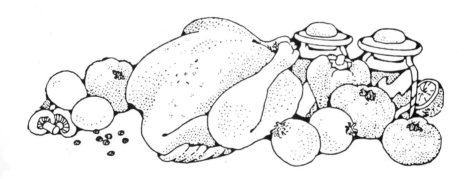

Fish

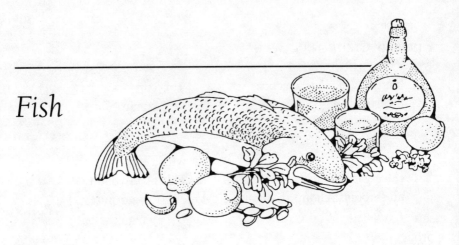

Fish is very delicate, and therefore deteriorates rapidly. It is difficult to judge its freshness from its appearance, since freezing methods can mask its age, but in general, the eyes of a fresh fish bulge and are bright, with a black pupil and transparent cornea; the gills are reddish pink; the scales adhere to the skin and have a sheen to them; the odor of the fish is non-offensive, especially around the gills or belly, but smells something like seaweed. The flesh of the fish is firm to the touch and bounces back when you touch it, rather than forming an imprint. Fresh fish, when placed in cold water, will float rather than sink. The real criteria for freshness, however, are how it keeps after you buy it, its odor and appearance when you prepare it and, finally, of course, its taste.

For information on the best fish choices see Foods to Enjoy, p. 34.

Fish should be cooked quickly, since after a certain point (150°) the delicate tissues break down and the nutritious juices are lost. Broiling should never take longer than 10 minutes, and baking, at 375°, should take a maximum of ½ hour for a whole fish. Fish is generally done *before* the point at which it flakes easily with a fork.

FISH RECIPES

Quick Fish For One

¼ lb. filet of flounder or sole

2 Tbl. water

2 Tbl. soy sauce

1 inch ginger, minced

Put the fish in a low pyrex baking dish. Add enough water and soy sauce and ginger to just barely cover the fish. Put the dish into the broiler and broil approximately 5 minutes. While broiling, spoon some of the liquid mixture over the fish.

Optional:

Marinate the fish in the mixture for ½ hour before broiling.

Broiled Fish in Lemon Sauce (*Serves 4*)

1 lb. fish fillets such as scrod
   or sole

Sauce:

1 Tbl. butter

1 Tbl. olive oil

1 clove garlic, minced

1 Tbl. lemon juice

1 Tbl. chopped parsley

Note that other herbs, such as dill or tarragon in place of, or with parsley, are also delicious.

Wash the fish and pat dry. Put it into a pan which will fit in the broiler. Lightly sauté the garlic in the butter/oil mixture. Let cool slightly, then add the lemon juice and parsley. Brush both sides of the fish with the sauce, and broil 4–5 minutes on one side only.

FISH ORIENTALE (*Serves 4*)

1 lb. fish fillets, such as floun-   2 Tbl. water
   der, sole, or scrod.   ¼ c. soy sauce
2 Tbl. olive oil   2 scallions, chopped
4 slices fresh ginger

Heat the oil in a large fry pan. Add the fish, and cook till it is lightly brown on both sides. Drain most of the oil, then add soy sauce, scallions, water and ginger. Cover and simmer 5 minutes. Turn the fish and simmer another 5 minutes till done. Add a pinch of cayenne pepper, if you wish.

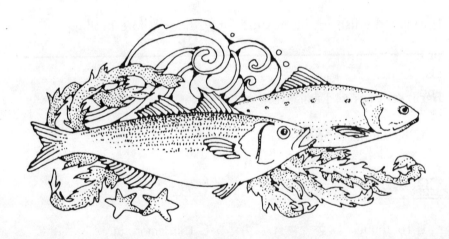

Vegetables: Entrées and Side Dishes

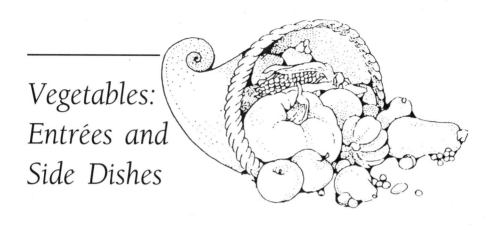

To get the most out of your vegetables, eat them raw, baked, grilled, or lightly steamed. Boiling vegetables destroys 20–45% of the minerals, 75% of the natural sugars, a large percentage of the vitamins, and all of the enzymes and life force. Enzyme destruction begins at 130°.

COOKING VEGETABLES

Vegetables, if cooked, should be steamed, baked, grilled or gently sautéed on a low heat in a little olive oil, canola oil, or butter.

Vegetables can also be made into wonderful soups.

Vegetables are done when they are slightly soft, but still have a crunchy texture and good color.

Most people find that rather than using specific recipes for cooking vegetables, they prefer to steam or sauté vegetables, or eat them raw, in various combinations that come to mind at the time of preparation, with ingredients that are easily available.

STEAMED VEGETABLES

Vegetables can be steamed together, or by themselves on a stainless steel, ceramic or bamboo steamer.

To steam most vegetables, bring the liquid under the steamer close to the boil, shut the heat off, cover the pot and let the vegetables cook in their own steam. It takes only minutes. This works especially well for the softer vegetables, although root vegetables will cook this way as well.

To steam especially hard vegetables, such as artichokes, bring the liquid under the steamer close to the boil, then turn it down to the lowest possible simmer, and let the vegetables cook, covered, till done.

Steaming vegetables over a broth instead of plain water adds a hint of flavor. Use miso broth, vegetable broth, soy sauce and water, or garlic and water.

Use spring or distilled water for steam water, then save it for a soup base or broth, or add it to sauces.

SAUTÉED VEGETABLES

Note: "Sauté" means lightly stirring on a low heat in a small amount of butter, canola oil, or olive oil. No frying, please!

Plan on about 2½ c. cut raw vegetables per serving. Cut in bite sized, thin slices to cook quickly and retain crispness.

Before sautéeing vegetables, separate them into three groups:

(1) onions and/or garlic
(2) harder, longer cooking vegetables, such as carrots, potatoes, green string beans, cauliflower
(3) softer, quick cookers such as zucchini, mushrooms, peppers, tomatoes

Put the vegetables in group (1) in the pan first, as they take the longest, then add those in group (2), then those in group (3).

One delicious, quick example is tomato-zucchini sauté. Sauté minced garlic, sliced zucchini and chopped tomatoes in olive oil till slightly soft. Add basil and/or grated parmesan cheese.

ADD TO SAUTÉED OR STEAMED VEGETABLES:

olive oil
butter or "better butter" (see p. 36)
soy sauce
lemon juice
canola oil
tofu or tahini sauce
ground nuts and seeds
sprouts
chopped parsley
minced garlic
cooked grain, noodles and/or beans
grated Parmesan cheese

CREATE-A-MEAL

The chart on the following page uses a fast and easy technique for creating whole meals using vegetables and any other foods, such as chicken, fish, whole grains, noodles or beans.

Simply steam your choice of ingredients over a broth in which other ingredients are cooking at the same time. When all ingredients are cooked (about 8 to 10 minutes), remove them from the steamer and from the steaming water. The ingredients can then be combined together or eaten separately. For example, if you cook noodles under the steamer and cook vegetables at the same time in the steamer, after they are cooked you can add the vegetables to the noodles, or eat them separately.

Top the cooked ingredients with a little olive oil, butter, soy sauce, miso/tahini sauce, or any other sauce of your choice.

This technique works especially well when cooking for one person, since small amounts fit well under the steamer.

Use these six different meal examples to stimulate your own ideas.

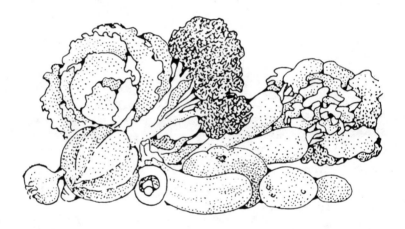

CREATE-A-MEAL IN A POT

These are quick, easy, delicious meals which serve 1. To make more, double the ingredients. Use this format to create your own recipes.

MEAL	POT INGREDIENTS	STEAMER INGREDIENTS	OPTIONAL SAUCE
Spicy Soba	1 oz. buckwheat soba noodles 2 c. water	1 small carrot, sliced 2 tsp. minced ginger ½ c. chopped tofu 3 Tbl. sliced mushrooms ½ c. snow peas 2 Tbl chopped almonds	Miso-tahini sauce with cayenne pepper added to taste
Sunchoke Pasta	1 oz. whole grain fettucini 2 c. water	1 c. diced cooked chicken ½ c. chopped sunchokes (Jerusalem artichokes) ½ c. fresh green peas ¼ c. sliced mushrooms	Miso-tahini sauce with tarragon added to taste (Use less miso than usual)
Poached Fish	4 oz. fish fillet 2 c. water	½ c. chopped broccoli ½ c. sliced leeks	Lemon juice, minced garlic and parsley
Vegetable Spaghetti	1 oz. whole grain spaghetti 2 c. water	1 c. sliced zucchini 1 c. chopped tomatoes ¼ c. chopped parsley	Tomato sauce and grated parmesen cheese
Ginger Fish & Veggies	1 oz. whole grain pasta 2 tsp. minced ginger 2 c. water	¾ c. diced raw fish (ex: haddock, cod) 1 small carrot, sliced ½ c. chopped broccoli ½ c. chopped cauliflower	Quick blended Super Sauce over the pasta, or over the combined ingredients
Fish 'n Rice	4 oz. fish fillet 2 c. water	1 c. cooked wild rice 3 Tbl. chopped almonds ¼ c. sliced leeks 2 Tbl. chopped parsley	Sprinkle with soy sauce

Directions:

Put the 2 c. water in a pot. Bring it close to a boil. Add the other "Pot Ingredients."

Turn the heat down to a low simmer. Put a vegetable steamer in the pot. Put the "Steamer Ingredients" into the steamer. Cover the pot.

Simmer on a low heat for 8 minutes. After 8 minutes, or when the vegetables are slightly soft, gently remove the steamer with the "steamer ingredients."

Strain the water off the "Pot Ingredients"—that is, off the pasta or fish.

You may now either combine the steamer ingredients with the pot ingredients (the pasta or fish), or eat them separately.

Use the "Optional Sauce" over the combined or separated ingredients.

RECIPES FOR VEGETABLE ENTRÉES AND SIDE DISHES

QUICK VEGETABLE CASSEROLE

Steamed or baked vegetables can be mixed or blended with an egg, melted butter and any spices, and, if you like, cooked grain. Then, lightly oil a casserole dish, put the mixture in the dish and bake. For example, add cooked broccoli to the rice-nut-cheese loaf, p. 230.

Or, put the pre-cooked mixture in a pre-made pie crust for a vegetable pie. See sweet potato scallion pie, p. 214.

VEGETABLE FOO YUNG (Serves 4)

2 Tbl. sesame oil	8–10 oz. tofu, in chunks
1 onion, finely chopped	½ c. sliced water chestnuts
1 clove garlic, minced	¼ c. soaked Chinese
2 Tbl. sesame seeds	mushrooms
2 c. shredded Chinese cabbage	¼ c. mung bean sprouts
1 c. snow peas	

Slightly heat the oil in a fry pan. Add the garlic, onion and sesame seeds and sauté till the onion is transparent. Add all ingredients but the sprouts and stir till slightly soft. Add sprouts and soy sauce to taste.

FLOUR-FREE VEGETABLE PIE (*Serves 6*)

3 large potatoes, sliced thin (no more than ¼" thick)
1 Tbl. butter
3 Tbl. olive oil
1 clove garlic, minced
2 medium zucchini, sliced thin

¼ tsp. each: basil and oregano
2 ripe tomatoes, sliced thin
a mixture of ½ c. grated swiss cheese and ½ c. grated Parmesan or goat cheese

Preheat the oven to 400°.
Melt the butter in a pan. Add the garlic.
Dip the potato slices in the garlic butter.
Line the bottom and sides of a 9" pie plate with one layer of potato. Put one layer of zucchini on top of the potato, layering to the edge of the plate. Sprinkle the herbs on top of the zucchini. Add a layer of tomato, then the cheese.
Bake at 400° until the potatoes are crispy and the cheese is browned (about 1 hour).

ALL-AMERICAN PIZZA

Use a whole grain English muffin*

Amounts per muffin half

one slice of tomato
⅛ tsp. minced garlic
pinch dried oregano and basil

¼ tsp. olive oil
1 Tbl. grated hard cheese
⅛ tsp. grated Parmesan

Lightly toast the muffin. Top with a slice of tomato, the garlic and spices, then the oil and cheese. Bake at 350° until the cheese is melted and the tomato soft.

*NOTE: For a large pizza, use a large whole grain bialy or pita bread.

SUNBURGERS

There are many varieties of nut burgers. Experiment on your own, using different kinds of vegetables and nuts and seeds.

Sunburgers can be eaten raw, as well as cooked. Just use less onion and garlic.

Top sunburgers with tomato sauce or sugarfree ketchup or tomato sauce.

In a pinch, sunburgers freeze well.

Suggested ingredients for sunburgers:

(These ingredients make about 6 burgers:)

1½ c. freshly ground sunflower seeds (about 1 c. unground seeds)

2 Tbl. chopped onions (small pieces)

1 clove garlic, minced

½ c. grated carrots (about 1 medium carrot)

½ c. chopped celery (about 1 large stalk)

1 Tbl. chopped parsley

2 tsp. chopped green pepper

2 Tbl. wheat germ

⅛ tsp. basil

½ tsp. soy sauce

1 egg, beaten

1 Tbl. sesame or olive oil

¼ c. tomato juice, or water

Sunburger preparation:

Mix sunflower seed meal, vegetables and spices, except the soy sauce.

In a separate bowl, mix the beaten egg, oil and soy sauce, then add that to the vegetable mixture.

Thoroughly combine the two mixtures, then add juice or water to make a doughy consistency.

Shape into patties and arrange on an oiled baking sheet.

At 350° bake 15 minutes on one side, then turn the patties and bake 10 minutes more.

Blended Sunburgers:

If you have a strong blender, the ingredients for the sunburger can be chopped and mixed in the blender.

Grind the seeds, put them aside, then add the carrots, celery and green pepper (which have been chopped slightly) and the rest of the ingredients. Blend well, then add to the sunflower meal.

RAW FERMENTED SEED LOAF

3 c. ground sesame seeds
3 c. ground sunflower seeds
1 c. ground almonds
1 green pepper, chopped
1 onion, chopped
2 stalks celery, chopped

3 cloves garlic, minced
1 c. parsley, chopped
1 Tbl. basil and 1 tsp. thyme
½ tsp. each oregano and marjoram
pinch cumin

Optional:

1 tsp. powdered kelp, and/or, 1 to 2 Tbl. soy sauce.

Mix the ingredients in a large bowl. Add enough water or rejuvelac (fermented grain water—see p. 154) to make a dough. You will need only about 2 to 3 Tbl. liquid, since the loaf becomes much more moist as it ferments. It is better to use rejuvelac, since the enzymes in the rejuvelac help digest the heavy protein of the nuts and seeds.

Leave the loaf in a warmish place, or at room temperature for 24 to 28 hours. Cover it with a damp cloth to keep it from drying out. The longer it sits, the more fermented it will become, and the tangier the taste.

Serving Suggestion:

Halve a green pepper, remove the seeds and put a small amount of seed loaf inside. Top with a slice of tomato and a sprig of parsley. Or, spread the loaf on crackers with parsley, tomato and sprouts.

Please Note: Eat *small* amounts, no more than ½ c. at a time. It's very concentrated.

SWEET POTATO SCALLION PIE

Crust:

¾ c. brown rice flour   ⅓ c. butter, slightly soft
½ c. oat flour   3 Tbl. ice water

Preheat the oven to 400°.
Lightly oil a 9" pie pan.

Combine the flours in a large bowl. With a pastry blender, cut the butter into the flour till you have pea sized crumbles. Sprinkle in the ice water, mixing briefly with a fork.

Form the mixture into a ball.

Lightly flour a piece of wax paper larger than 11" round. Also flour a rolling pin.

Roll out a circle of the mixture, about ¼" thick and 10½" round, onto the wax paper. Gently unroll the wax paper from the dough circle, placing the dough in the pie pan.

Flute the edges, if you wish.

Prick the bottom of the crust in several places with a fork.

Bake at 400° for 10 to 12 minutes, or until it just begins to turn lightly brown.

Filling:

1 Tbl. melted butter	½ c. soy or nut milk, or water
1 Tbl. olive oil	½ c. water
¼ c. chopped scallions	
1 egg	
2 c. cooked sweet potato (2 large sweet potatoes—approximately 1¼ lb.)	

Heat the butter and oil in a small fry pan. Lightly sauté the scallions.

Beat the egg in a large bowl, or blender. Add the cooked sweet potatoes, milk, water and butter/scallion mixture. Beat with an electric beater, or blend in a strong blender till smooth. Pour the filling into the crust and bake at 400° for 45 minutes to 1 hour.

BAKED SQUASH WITH WILD RICE STUFFING

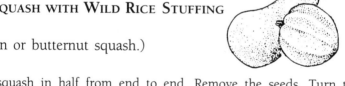

(Use acorn or butternut squash.)

Slice the squash in half from end to end. Remove the seeds. Turn the squash face down on a lightly oiled pan. (This keeps it from drying out.) Bake at 350° for 45 minutes. Meanwhile, prepare the stuffing.

Stuffing:

1 Tbl. butter	⅔ c. whole grain bread cubes
1 Tbl. olive oil	3 tsp. dried parsley
1 clove garlic, minced	1 tsp. dried thyme
1 Tbl. chopped onion	¾ c. cooked wild rice
⅔ c. chopped mushrooms	⅓ c. chopped celery

Crush the dried parsley and thyme in a mortar or cup.

Sauté the minced garlic, chopped onions and mushroom in the

butter. Add the bread cubes and crushed herbs. Stir well till combined, then add the rice and celery. Mix.

Makes enough to fill the cavities of both halves of the squash.

After the squash bakes face down for 45 minutes, turn it face up and fill the cavities with the stuffing. Bake another 15 to 20 minutes.

Alternative to the stuffing:

For a sweet alternative to the stuffing, fill the cavities with a pat of butter and 2 Tbl. gingered carrot marmalade (see p. 197).

SUPER EASY SIDE DISHES

TOMATOES PROVENCAL *(Serves 4)*

4 ripe tomatoes	1 Tbl. grated Parmesan cheese
2 tsp. basil	1½ Tbl. olive oil
1 tsp. oregano	½ tsp. butter
2 cloves garlic, minced	
¼ lb. Swiss cheese, grated, or mozzarella, sliced	

Optional:

Powdered kelp or cayenne pepper added after cooking.

Slice the tomatoes in half. Put them in a lightly oiled baking dish. Sprinkle the tomatoes with basil and oregano, then with the Swiss and Parmesan cheese.

In a small pan, melt the butter on a low heat, then add the olive oil and minced garlic. Sprinkle this mixture over the tomatoes.

Bake at 350° for 45 minutes.

PORT SALUT NOODLE CASSEROLE

Prep Time: 15 minutes   **Cook Time: 10 minutes**

30ml	(2 tbsp.) olive oil	30ml	(2 tbsp.) minced fresh basil, divided
1	small onion, minced	30ml	(2 tbsp.) salt
1	clove garlic, minced	30ml	(2 tbsp.) pepper
473ml	(2 cups) sliced shiitake mushroom caps	227g	(8 oz.) egg noodles, cooked
1	(793g/28-oz.) can crushed tomatoes	237ml	(1 cup) thinly sliced Port Salut cheese

1. Preheat oven to 163°C/325°F. Grease a 22.86 centimetre (9-inch)-square ovenproof glass baking dish. Heat oil in large skillet over medium-high heat. Add onion and garlic. Cook 1 minute. Add mushrooms and cook for 3 to 4 minutes, stirring frequently. Add crushed tomatoes, 22 millilitres (1½ tablespoons) of the basil, salt and pepper. Cook 5 minutes. Stir in cooked egg noodles and heat through.

2. Spoon noodle mixture into baking dish. Combine remaining 7.5 millilitres (½ tablespoon) basil and cheese. Arrange over noodles. Bake 10 minutes or until cheese melts.

Serves 4

Recipe Note: If desired, use crushed tomatoes with Italian seasoning blend and skip the garlic.

Per Serving: 470 calories/kJ-, 19g protein, 54g carbohydrate, 6g dietary fibre, 19g fat (36% of calories from fat), 80mg cholesterol, 282.88mg potassium, 650mg sodium, .21g Omega-3

Port Salut Noodle Casserole

SHIITAKE MUSHROOM

SWEET POTATO PUDDING

1 cooked sweet potato
1 egg
1 Tbl. butter

Nutmeg, cinnamon and/or allspice to taste

Blend well in a blender. Add water if this is too thick.
Some people love this for breakfast.

HERBED POTATO

Slice a baking potato in half, leaving the jacket on. Butter it lightly
on the cut end. Place it in a pan, cut end down, on a thin bed of
caraway or cumin seeds. Bake at 350° till done (about 45 minutes).

POTATO PANCAKES (*Makes 12 pancakes*)

½ c. chopped onions
2½ c. grated potato (approxi-
    mately 1 lb. mature potatoes)

2 tsp. soy sauce
2 eggs
2 Tbl. brown rice flour

Sauté the onions in butter, till lightly browned.

Put the grated potato in a clean white cotton cloth or cheese
cloth. Thoroughly squeeze out the excess moisture. (You may need
to press a small amount of potato at a time. If you use cheese cloth,
you can rinse it out afterwards and use it again.)

Beat the eggs in a large bowl. Add the soy sauce, onions and
potato. Mix well, then add the flour and mix again.

Form patties of the mixture. Cook them in butter or olive oil in
a fry pan till lightly browned. You will need to turn them.

Serve with plain yogurt, kefir cheese or homemade apple sauce.

STEAMED ARTICHOKE

Choose an artichoke that is fairly tight without any brown spots and that "squeaks" when you gently squeeze it. Cut off the stem. Pull off the tough bottom row of leaves and, if you like, cut off the prickly tips with scissors.

Place the artichoke upright on a steamer. Bring the water to the lowest possible simmer, and cover the pot. Steam for about 45 minutes till the leaves pull off easily.

Drain and serve hot or cold.

Artichoke Sauce:

Use a traditional hollandaise sauce, or mix melted butter and lemon juice, and, if you like, minced garlic.

STEAMED GARLIC BROCCOLI *(Serves 1–2)*

¾ c. broccoli flowerettes   1 clove garlic, minced
¼ c. sliced broccoli stem
¾ c. sliced leek (the white part
    and the tender green part)

Steam the broccoli stems. When slightly soft, add the flowerettes, the leek and the minced garlic. Steam till slightly soft.

Suggested Additions:

Melted butter or olive oil and/or lemon juice and/or soy sauce.

Grains

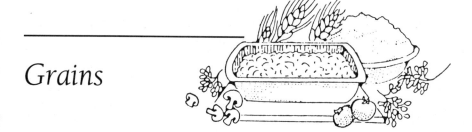

Use only whole, unprocessed, unrefined grains. Refined grains have been stripped of almost all nutrients—vitamin E, protein, B vitamins and other vitamins and minerals, as well as fiber, so necessary for good health.

Keep grains (as well as flour, nuts, seeds, and oils) in the refrigerator or freezer to avoid rancidity and bug infestation.

Grains can be sprouted, cooked ground or whole, eaten as cereals, side dishes, in casseroles, patties, soups, sauces, broths, or in various mixtures with other grains, beans, vegetables and nuts and seeds.

All grains should be rinsed in cold water before cooking in order to remove excess starch and grit and to begin the swelling process. Put the grain in a large pot. Add enough tap water to cover. Swirl the grain around. Drain. Repeat if necessary until the water is clear.

Remember that in soaking or cooking grains, they increase in volume, so use a pot large enough to accommodate the increase. Use a non-aluminum pot with a tight fitting lid, as the grains should cook in their own steam.

Use approximately ¼–½ cup dry grain per person. For a side dish or for breakfast, ½–¾ cup cooked grain per person is sufficient, and for a main course, 1 cup cooked grain per person.

Sometimes you will come across a difference in grain hybrids, such as short grain or long grain rice. Short grain will come out tender and moist, and is best for most recipes. Long grain is better in recipes for rice stuffing, or for soups.

Cook grains slowly on as low heat as possible to preserve the most nutritional value and life force. To help you cook on a low heat, use a flame tamer or bent wire between the pot and the flame.

To avoid mushy grains, do not stir except where indicated. Once the pot lid is on and the grains are cooking, try not to peek until the cooking time is up.

Grains are ready to eat when they are chewy, and not overly soft or too hard. If you want a porridge, blend the cooked grain with a liquid and, if you like, soaked dried fruit, nuts or seeds, soy sauce, tahini, or miso.

The preparation of grains can spark much creativity by combining them with various ingredients listed below. Though it is always best to eat freshly cooked grain, some people find it makes life easier when they keep some cooked grain handy in the refrigerator, where it will keep for three to four days.

Leftover grain can be made into creamy cereals, breads, salads, sauces, soups, or grain broths. Or, lightly sautée cooked grains in olive oil and garlic with freshly steamed or raw vegetables, nuts and seeds, or cooked beans or noodles.

Combining grains with beans and tofu, sauces made from beans or tofu, or with nuts and seeds increases the protein availability. Delicious sauces can be made with tahini, miso or tofu.

VARIATIONS OF INGREDIENTS IN COOKING GRAIN:

LIQUID BASES:

Cook the grain in any of the following:

    water
    vegetable stock
    nut milk

soy milk

vegetable juice

miso stock

herb tea (Cooking grains in teas such as peppermint, oatstraw or chamomile may aid in the digestion and assimilation as well as adding a different flavor.)

MIX TOGETHER BEFORE COOKING:

Good combinations of grains that have similar cooking time are:

> rye + rice   rice + wheat
> rye + oats   rice flakes + oat flakes
> rye + barley   rice + millet
> mix with:
> wheat germ
> nuts and seeds, ground or whole
> rehydrated (soaked) dried fruit

ADD TO COOKED GRAINS AFTER COOKING FOR TASTE & NUTRITIONAL VARIATION:

steamed or raw vegetables

sautéed onions, scallions, leeks or garlic

soaked seaweed

ground nuts and seeds

cooked noodles

cooked beans

sprouts

sauce: tofu, tahini-ginger, "super sauce," miso/tahini, tomato, etc.

butter, olive oil or sesame oil

soy sauce

nutritional yeast

cayenne pepper

chopped parsley

minced ginger

spices and herbs. Whole cloves, a stick of cinnamon or a bay leaf can be added to the cooking grain to add a hint of flavor. Remove the herb before eating. Herbs and spices can be added after cooking, as well.

vanilla extract

honey

molasses

GRAIN COOKING TECHNIQUES

There are several ways to cook grains, depending on the type of grain and on the method that is easiest for you at the time. Whenever possible, aim for the method that uses the lowest possible heat.

"Simmer" and "pilaf" methods are good, but they require the most heat.

"Soak and Simmer" or "Double Boiler" methods are better, since they use less heat.

"Soak and Steam," "Thermos" or "Quick Steam" are best, since they require the least amount of heat.

When you choose a method, naturally you will need to consider what is most practical for you as well.

See the *Grain Cooking Chart* on page 224 for a listing of grains, their cooking methods, amounts and cooking time.

QUICK STEAM

There are two ways to quick-steam grains, depending on the type of grain.

1. For buckweat, roasted buckweat (kasha) and bulgur (cracked wheat):

Put the grain in a pot.
In a separate pot, bring the liquid close to a boil, then pour it over the grain.
Stir the grain once.
Cover the pot with a tightly fitting lid.
Let stand, covered till done (about 10 to 15 minutes).

2. For rolled oats: Cooking buckwheat or bulgur with this method works, but the grain gets a little mushy.

Put the grain and the liquid in a pot. Bring the liquid close to a boil. Stir the grain once. Cover the pot. Shut off the heat and let the grain cook in its own steam till done (about 10 minutes).

SOAK & STEAM

For wild rice, brown rice, barley, millet, rye, wheat, triticale:
Soak the grain in the necessary amount of liquid (see page 224) for 36 hours.
After soaking the grain, add more liquid, if necessary, so that you have the same amount of liquid as grain. (For example, for ½ c. soaked grain, you will need ½ c. liquid.)
Bring the soaked grain and the liquid close to a boil.
Shut off the heat.
Cover the pot and let the grain cook in its own steam for approximately 4 to 5 hours, or until done. If it is more convenient, let it steam all day, or overnight. You may need to bring it to the boil again after a few hours.
For example, begin to soak the grain at 8 PM Friday night. Soak time will be completed at 8 AM Sunday morning. Then let the grain sit in its own steam all day Sunday, or at least 4 to 5 hours.
Or, begin the soaking process at 8 AM Friday. Soaking will be

GRAIN COOKING CHART

COOKING METHOD & TIME

GRAIN	DRY GRAIN AMOUNT	AMOUNT OF LIQUID	QUICK STEAM	SOAK & STEAM	SOAK & SIMMER	DOUBLE BOILER	THERMOS	LOW SIMMER	PILAF	COOKED GRAIN AMOUNT
Amaranth	1 c.	3 c.		36 hrs. + 4 hrs.	12 hrs. + 15 min.	35 min.	12 hrs.	20 min.	25 min.	3 c.
Barley	1/2 c.	1 1/2 c.		36 hrs. + 4 hrs.	12 hrs. + 10 min.	45 min.	12 hrs.	30 min.	30 min.	2 c.
Buckwheat	1 c.	1 1/4 c.	10–15 min.			15 min.	10 min.	5 min.	5 min.	2 1/4 c
Bulgur	1/2 c.	1 c.	10–15 min.			15 min.	10 min.	5 min.	5 min.	1 1/2 c.
Cornmeal*	1/2 c.	2 1/2 c.				30 min.			30 min.	3 c.
Millet	1/2 c.	1 1/2 c.		36 hrs. + 4 hrs.	12 hrs. + 10 min.	35 min.	12 hrs.	20 min.	35 min.	2 c.
Oats	1/2 c.	2 c.		36 hrs. + 5 hrs.	12 hrs. + 15 min.	60 min.	12 hrs.	45 min.	45 min.	1 1/2 c.
Rolled Oats*	1 c.	2 1/2 c.	10 min.			15 min.	10 min.			2 c.
Quinoa	1 c.	2 c.	25 min.	36 hrs. + 4 hrs.	12 hrs. + 15 min.	15 min.	15 min.	20 min.	20 min.	3 c.

Cooking Method & Time

Grain	Dry Grain Amount	Amount of Liquid	Quick Steam	Soak & Steam	Soak & Simmer	Double Boiler	Thermos	Low Simmer	Pilaf	Cooked Grain Amount
Brown Rice	¾ c.	1½ c.		36 hrs. + 5 hrs.	12 hrs. + 15 min.	45 min.	8 hrs.	30 min.	30 min.	2 c.
Wild Rice	½ c.	1¾ c.		36 hrs. + 5 hrs.	12 hrs. + 15 min.	90 min.	12 hrs.	60 min.	60 min.	2 c.
Rice Flour**	¼ c.	1 c.				30 min.				2 c.
Rye	½ c.	2 c.		36 hrs. + 5 hrs.	12 hrs. + 15 min.	90 min.	12 hrs.	60 min.	60 min.	1½ c.
Rye Flakes	1 c.	2½ c.	10 min.			15 min.	10 min.			2 c.
Triticale	½ c.	2 c.		36 hrs. + 5 hrs.	12 hrs. + 10 min.	60 min.	12 hrs.	45 min.	50 min.	1⅓ c.
Wheat	½ c.	2 c.		36 hrs. + 5 hrs.	12 hrs. + 10 min.	60 min.		45 min.	50 min.	1⅓ c.

* See "Cereals."

** Any grain can be ground to a flour and prepared as a Cream Cereal. See "Cereals".

READING THIS CHART:

This chart shows the cook time for 7 different methods of cooking grains, along with the dry grain amount, required liquid amount, and the amount of cooked grain.

completed 8 PM Saturday. Let the grain steam-cook overnight Saturday. It will be ready Sunday morning.

The soaked grain will keep refrigerated in its soak liquid up to one week if you do not wish to begin the steaming process right away.

SOAK & SIMMER

For wild rice, brown rice, barley, millet, rye, wheat, triticale—whole or ground:

12 hours before eating time, bring the grain and the liquid close to the boil, then shut the heat off, cover the pot, and let the grain cook in its own steam for 12 hours (overnight or all day).

Just before eating, bring the grain and liquid close to the boil again, turn the heat down to the lowest possible simmer, and simmer until done (about 10–15 minutes).

THERMOS COOKED GRAIN

For wild rice, brown rice, barley, millet, whole rye, triticale. Other grains such as buckwheat, rolled oats and rye flakes can be cooked with this method but they may be too soft. Wheat cooked this way becomes rubbery. If your thermos does not hold heat well, this technique will not work.

Use a one quart wide mouthed thermos. Add the grain and any other ingredients (nuts and seeds, dried fruit, etc.), then the required amount of liquid or broth which has been heated just to the boiling point.

With the handle of a long wooden spoon, stir the grain to distribute the liquid evenly.

(Do not fill water right up to the top. Allow at least 1 inch from the top.)

Screw the lid on tightly and let stand 8 to 12 hours.

Grains can be put into the thermos whole or ground. If you want a creamy cereal, blend it after it is cooked.

PILAF METHOD

For barley, buckwheat or kasha, bulgur, millet, oats, brown rice, wild rice, rye, triticale, wheat:

Sauté onions and/or garlic in oil in a pan that has a lid. Add the grain and, if you like, nuts and seeds. Sauté on a low heat, then add a liquid such as water, vegetable or miso stock. Cook on the lowest possible heat till nearly done, then add chopped vegetables. Cover the pan and turn the heat off so that the vegetables cook in their own steam.

LOW SIMMER

For barley, millet, oats, brown rice, wild rice, rye, triticale, wheat:

Bring the grain and liquid close to the boil, then turn the heat down to the lowest possible setting. If possible, use a flame-tamer between the pot and the flame. Stir the grain once, cover the pot and let it gently cook for the required amount of time. Try not to peek until the cook time is up. Otherwise, the grain tends to get mushy.

DOUBLE BOILER

For all grains. Cornmeal, rice cream and other ground grains cook best this way.

Fill the bottom half of the double boiler about ⅓ to ½ full with tap water. Bring that water to a gentle simmer and leave the pot on the burner.

Meanwhile, fill the top half of the double boiler with the required amount of grain-cooking liquid and place that pot directly over another burner. Bring that liquid close to a boil, then turn it down to a gentle simmer. Slowly pour in the grain meal, stirring constantly with a wire whisk to avoid lumping. When the grain meal has absorbed the liquid, cover the pot and put it over the bottom half of the double boiler, which is still at a low simmer. Let cook till done.

If you are cooking a cereal, you can save a little time in the morning by soaking the grain overnight in the hot liquid:

Bring the ground grain (plus raisins or other dried fruit) and the liquid (water or nut milk) close to the boil, shut the heat off, cover the pot and let it sit overnight. In the morning, bring the grain and liquid close to the boil again, then put it over the double boiler and "cook" about 10 to 15 minutes.

GRAIN RECIPES

BROWN RICE (*Makes 2 c. grain*)

½ c. raw brown rice   1 c. water

Rinse the rice until the rinse water is clear. Drain. Bring the rice
and water close to a boil. Turn the heat to the lowest possible
setting. Stir once. Tightly cover the pot. Cook gently ½ hour. Try
not to peek. If after the ½ hour, the rice is just the tiniest bit soggy,
cover the pot, turn off the heat, and let sit 10 minutes. Don't stir
it. It will continue to cook in its own heat.

MILLET (*Makes 2 c. cooked grain*)

½ c. millet   2 c. water

Rinse the millet till the rinse water is clear. Drain. Bring the millet
and water close to the boil. Turn the heat to the lowest possible
setting. Tightly cover the pot and cook 20 minutes.

RICE-NUT-CHEESE LOAF (*Serves 4*)

2 c. cooked brown rice

1 clove garlic, minced

½ c. chopped onion (1 medium sized onion)

1 c. chopped walnuts

¼ tsp. soy sauce

2 eggs, beaten or 1 egg + 2 egg whites

¾ lb. sharp cheddar cheese, grated

½ c. water or soy milk

Mix all ingredients. Put them into a lightly greased 9" x 5" or 10" x 6" casserole. Bake for 50 to 60 minutes at 350°. Let sit 10 minutes before cutting.

This makes a great leftover—not as rich as it is when just cooked and hot.

Alternate:

Add ¾ c. cooked vegetables to the other ingredients before baking.

SESAME RICE (*Serves 2*)

2 tsp. butter or sesame oil

⅓ c. sliced leeks or scallions

1½ Tbl. sesame seeds

2 c. cooked brown rice

Optional: ¼ tsp. soy sauce, or to taste

Lightly sauté on a low heat the leeks or scallions, and sesame seeds in the butter or oil. Add the rice, and stir till warm and mixed with the other ingredients. Add soy sauce to taste, if you like. This is also great with tahini gravy or "super sauce."

PILAF CASSEROLE *(Serves 3–4)*

1 Tbl. olive oil
3 Tbl. chopped onion (about 1 small onion)
½ c. chopped mushrooms (2–3 large mushrooms)
1 c. uncooked grain—bulgur, buckwheat, rice or millet, or a mixture of them

2 Tbl. chopped green pepper
1 Tbl. chopped parsley
½ c. chopped celery
1 small carrot, chopped
2 to 4 c. vegetable stock and 1 Tbl. soy sauce, or use miso broth.

Optional:

add ½ tsp. sage or cumin

Preheat the oven to 350°.

Heat the oil in a one quart casserole. Lightly sauté the onion, mushrooms, and grain, then add the stock and any spices. The amount of broth depends on the type of grain used in the recipe. Refer to the suggestions on the following page, and to the Grain Cooking Chart (p. 224–5) to determine how much liquid to add for the grain you choose.

Bring the liquid just to the boil, stir, cover and reduce the heat to the lowest possible temperature. Gently simmer 15 minutes.

Add the vegetables. Put the casserole in the oven and bake, covered, at 350° for 30–40 minutes, or until all the liquid is absorbed and the grain is dry, yet tender.

Suggested combinations for the Pilaf Casserole:

After sautéing the onion in olive oil, add any of the following combinations and bake as indicated:

• 1 c. bulgur plus sesame seeds, cumin and raisins in 2 c. vegetable stock.

- ⅓ c. each millet and lentils with bay leaf, sage, lovage in 4 c. vegetable broth.
- 1 c. brown rice plus curry powder, cumin, walnuts, bay leaf, in 2 ½ c. water.
- 1 c. bulgur plus garlic and dill in 2 c. tomato juice.
- 1 c. brown rice plus walnuts in 2 c. miso broth.
- ¾ c. millet plus sage in 3 c. vegetable broth.

WILD RICE 'N PASTA

¼ c. cooked wild rice	2 Tbl. chopped parsley
¼ c. cooked Jerusalem artichoke spaghetti	2 Tbl. sliced green leek
6 almonds, chopped	1 Tbl. butter/olive oil combination
¼ c. soft tofu	2 tsp. soy sauce
1–2 Tbl. sliced celery	

Lightly sauté the almonds and leeks in the butter in a fry pan. Add all other ingredients and stir till warm. Add the soy sauce last, to taste.

This serves one person with a good appetite. Increase the amounts for serving more than one.

QUINOA/POTATO CROQUETTES

2 cups quinoa, cooked	1 tsp. olive oil
2 cups potato, cooked (mashed with skins on)	½ tsp. rosemary
1 egg, beaten	½ tsp. salt

Combine ingredients. Form into patties. Place on lightly oiled baking sheet. Bake at 450° for 15 minutes on a side.

QUINOA PIE CRUST

¾ cup quinoa, rinsed   ¼ cup olive or canola oil
¼ cup boiling water   pinch salt (optional)

Put the quinoa in a blender and blend until ground into flour. Put the flour in a medium size bowl and mix in the salt.

Put the boiling water and oil in the blender. Blend until the mixture is white and frothy.

Add the oil-water mixture to the flour and stir until all liquid is blended in.

Press the dough into a lightly oiled shallow 9-inch pie pan.

Add the pie ingredients to the unbaked crust and bake in a preheated oven at 350°.

GRAIN SALADS

QUICK GRAIN SALAD (Serves 1)

Prepare ½ c. strong peppermint tea. While it is steeping, mix the following:

½ c. bulgur (cracked wheat)   1 Tbl. currants
2 Tbl. sunflower seeds

Pour the tea over the above mixture and let it sit till the grain is soft (about 10 minutes). When the grain has absorbed the tea, add chopped parsley.

Note: Bulgur is wheat. If you are allergic to wheat, use unroasted buckwheat or roasted buckwheat (kasha). Add more tea if you prefer a softer texture; otherwise, the buckwheat will be crunchy.

Optional additions:
These additions make the salad slightly more elaborate, but don't add that much time to the preparation.

To the steeped peppermint tea, add:

2 tsp. lemon juice   ½ tsp. soy sauce
¼ tsp. cinnamon

To the salad, after soaking, add:

1 Tbl. chopped scallions   ½ ripe tomato, diced

MOCK TABOULI (BULGUR SALAD)

This is a recipe that is easy to prepare ahead for a large party. It keeps very well, up to one week refrigerated.

Also note that this recipe requires no cooking, other than boiling water!

Ingredients for 8 portions:

Combine:

2 c. bulgur wheat   ¾ c. sunflower seeds
   water to cover grain (about   ¾ c. currants
   1½ to 2 c.)   ½ c. chopped parsley
2 peppermint tea bags   ⅓ c. chopped scallions

Optional:

½ c. chopped fresh mint; sliced tomatoes; chopped cucumber

Dressing:

⅓ c. + 1 Tbl. olive oil   2½ Tbl. lemon juice
¼ c. soy sauce   ½ tsp. minced garlic
¼ tsp. cinnamon

Ingredients for 50 portions:

10 c. bulgur	3 qts. water
6 peppermint tea bags	3 c. currants
2½ c. sunflower seeds	3 c. chopped parsley
3 c. chopped scallions	2 c. chopped mint

Dressing (Make more if you prefer a more moist salad):

⅔ c. lemon juice	⅔ c. soy sauce
1½ c. olive oil	½ Tbl. cinnamon
¾ Tbl. powdered garlic	

Mock Tabouli Preparation:

Steep the tea bags in the water until you have a strong peppermint tea.

Put the bulgur in a bowl, allowing about 3" from the top of the bowl so that the bulgur can rise as it soaks up the tea. Pour enough tea over the bulgur so that the grain is wet, but there is no tea above the level of the grain. Put a plate on top of the bulgur so that the top will not dry out. Soak for one hour, or until the grain has absorbed all the tea.

While the bulgur is soaking, put the sunflower seeds and currants in one bowl, the vegetables in another bowl, and the dressing in another bowl.

When the bulgur is soft, mix a small amount of bulgur together with small amounts of seed-currant mixture, vegetables and dressing, transferring the mixed tabouli to a separate bowl. This helps keep the tabouli light and fluffy. (This is especially necessary when making larger amounts.)

If the tabouli is drier than you prefer, add more dressing.

Decorate with cherry tomatoes, sprigs of parsley, and lettuce leaves around the edges.

WILD RICE SALAD WITH CURRIED TOFU MAYONNAISE
(Makes 4½ cups of salad)

Combine:

1 c. cooked brown rice	2 Tbl. chopped celery leaves
1¾ c. cooked wild rice	1 Tbl. chopped parsley
3 Tbl. slivered almonds	½ c. chopped apple
¾ c. chopped celery	

Optional:

Add ¼ c. raisins

CURRIED TOFU MAYONNAISE *(Makes 1⅓ c.)*

Blend well in a blender till smooth:

8 oz. firm tofu	¼ tsp. soy sauce
2 Tbl. cider vinegar	1 tsp. curry powder
2 Tbl. olive oil	4 to 5 Tbl. water
½ tsp. mustard	

Pasta

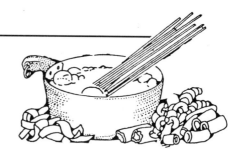

Use whole grain, unrefined, unprocessed pasta. Especially tasty are whole wheat, 100% buckwheat (which is not wheat), and those made with a combination of Jerusalem artichoke flour and whole wheat. There is also wheat free pasta for those allergic to wheat, made from rye or rice flour, corn flour, quinoa flour, and other new non-allergenic grains.

In general follow the cooking instructions on the package. Bring the water to a gently rolling boil, and add the pasta gradually so that the boil is not disturbed. You can hold the noodles on one end, and, while they soften, slowly push them down into the hot water.

To help keep the noodles from clumping, add a little olive oil to the cooking water. Also, to help cut the starchy covering of noodles, put the cooking water aside after you drain the noodles, rinse the drained noodles in cold water, then put them back in the cooking water for a second to re-warm them.

Pasta is fun to experiment with and to create your own spontaneous recipes.

Pasta is delicious as a side dish with a sauce, in cold salads, or added to soups, lightly sautéed vegetables, or grains.

Having pasta at the same meal with legumes (beans), or a bean by-product, such as miso or tofu, makes the usable protein more complete.

PASTA

PASTA & SAUCE

Cooked pasta is delicious with any of the following sauces or dressings:

- Olive oil, minced garlic and parsley
- Butter and soy sauce
- Butter or olive or sesame oil and chopped parsley
- Tomato sauce
- Super Sauce
- Miso-Tahini Sauce
- Sesame Tahini Sauce
- Tahini-Ginger Dressing
- Quick Lentil Sauce
- Oil and Vinegar Dressing
- Ruth Duffy's Dressing
- Mustard Dressing
- Tofu Dressing
- Curried Tofu Mayonnaise

PASTA PLUS

For an added treat, use a variety of pasta in the same dish—green
or white, fettucini or shells, etc.

While the pasta is cooking, sauté on a low heat in olive oil, or
canola oil, or butter any of the following:

onions   mushrooms
garlic   chopped leeks
chopped scallions   chopped peppers
chopped pecans, walnuts or almonds

Then add the pasta and any of the following:

cooked grain   cooked chicken or fish
steamed vegetables   cooked beans
chopped parsley   raw vegetables
ground or chopped nuts and seeds   sprouts
herbs and spices

Then, if you like, top that mixture with soy sauce or any of the
sauces listed on the left.

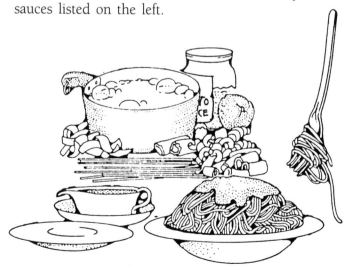

ITALIAN TOFU AND PASTA (*Serves 2*)

2 oz. whole wheat/Jerusalem artichoke flat fettucini

1 c. tofu pieces (firm tofu, cut
into ½" squares)

1 Tbl. fresh thyme or 1 tsp.
dried

2 Tbl. finely chopped fresh
parsley

1 large clove garlic, minced
(1 tsp.)

¼ c. olive oil

1 c. chopped tomatoes

Put a large pot of water on to boil.

Meanwhile, mix the thyme, parsley, garlic and olive oil in a pan that will fit under the broiler. Add the tofu pieces and stir thoroughly until the tofu is well covered with the mixture. Put the pan under the broiler to broil for 15 minutes. Stir the tofu occasionally.

Put the pasta into the boiling water and set the timer for the cook time indicated on the package (usually 8 minutes). Add 1 tsp. olive oil to the water to help keep the noodles from clumping.

When the pasta and tofu are done, add the drained noodles to the pan with the cooked tofu, stirring to cover the pasta with the oil and herb mixture.

Add the chopped tomatoes and stir again. Then transfer to a serving bowl.

This is delicious with a green salad, such as Avocado-Watercress or Watercress-Endive. (See pp. 176 and 178.)

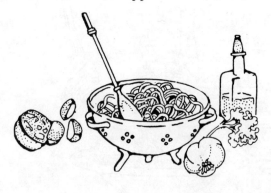

PECAN–PASTA SALAD (*Serves 2*)

1 c. medium whole wheat/Jerusalem artichoke pasta shells, cooked

1¼ c. sliced endive
1¼ c. watercress sprigs
14 pecans, chopped

Blend:

⅓ c. sesame oil
2 Tbl. cider vinegar
1 tsp. tarragon

¼ tsp. ground celery seed
1 clove garlic, minced (1 tsp.)
½ tsp. mustard

Combine the pasta, endive, watercress and pecans. Add about 2 Tbl. of the dressing to the mixture, and stir thoroughly. Add more dressing, if needed.

SUNCHOKE–NOODLES (*Serves 2*)

2 oz. buckwheat pasta
1 Tbl. sesame oil
3 Tbl. sliced leeks
¼ c. slices of Jerusalem artichoke

½ c. firm tofu chunks
¼ c. chopped parsley

Put the buckwheat pasta on to cook.

Put the sesame oil in a fry pan. Add the leeks. Gently sauté, then add the sunchokes and tofu, and stir till warm. Add the cooked noodles and parsley. Stir again.

Top with a quick mixture of tahini and soy sauce, or use Super Sauce, p. 194 or Tahini-Ginger Sauce, p. 187.

Beans & Tofu

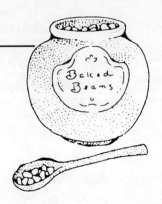

Many beans and peas can be sprouted and included in salads, or added to cooked dishes. All beans should be rinsed in cold water until the rinse water runs clear. Remove any stones or foreign particles.

All beans, except lentils, small limas, aduki beans, blackeyed peas and split peas should be soaked for at least three hours before cooking.

Remember that beans and peas expand greatly when soaking or cooking (2½ to 3 times), so use a pot with a tight fitting lid, large enough to accommodate the increase.

For smaller beans, such as lentils, split peas and limas, use about ¼ cup of dry beans per person for a serving. For other beans, use ½ c. dry beans per person.

As with grains, there are many variations in cooking liquids and in toppings for beans and peas.

For all legumes add two to four times more liquid than the volume of the legumes. Bring the liquid and the beans or peas just to the boil, cover the pot and turn the heat down to the lowest possible setting. Refer to the bean cooking chart, p. 245, for the required amount of liquid and cooking time for each type of bean.

Beans and peas must be cooked to prevent any toxic reaction that can occur from consuming raw beans (especially raw soy beans). However, low heat cooking is still preferable to a pressure cooker, since for most people beans will digest better if cooked on a low heat.

Some people find a crock pot works well for low heat cooking. Or, use your flame-tamer to help you cook on a low heat and avoid burning.

To help get rid of the carbohydrate that causes intestinal gas, throw out the soak water and add fresh water after each hour that the beans cook.

Adding a half of a potato or a teaspoon of apple cider vinegar to the cooking beans may also cut down on the gassy effect of the beans. The potato absorbs the gas-producing carbohydrate in the beans, and the vinegar aids the digestion.

Some people report that they have less gas from beans if they eat them at the same meal with rice.

Legumes (beans) can be eaten plain as a side dish, mixed with grains or vegetables, added to soups, or mashed as a spread or sauce.

LIQUIDS IN WHICH TO COOK BEANS:

Miso stock
Herb tea
Vegetable stock or juice
Water

ADD TO COOKED BEANS:

Nuts or seeds	Chopped parsley
Onions or garlic	Soy sauce
Cooked grain	Cooked pasta
Steamed vegetables	Raw vegetables

Sauces or dressings, such as olive oil, tofu sauce, tahini sauce, miso/tahini sauce, tomato sauce, or curried tofu mayonnaise.

SUGGESTED BEAN COMBINATIONS:

• Sauté onions and garlic in olive oil, add thyme and marjoram, then lentils, tomato and stock. Cook on a low simmer till nearly done (about ½ hour) then add chopped carrots and parsley.

• Cook aduki beans and butternut squash in water, miso stock or soy sauce.

• Bring split peas close to a boil. Reduce heat to the lowest possible simmer; add chopped onions. Cook till nearly soft (about 25 minutes), then add chopped carrots and cook 5 more minutes.

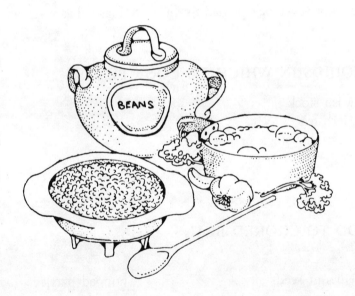

BEAN COOKING CHART

Unsoaked Beans (These do not need to be soaked)

BEAN	DRY BEANS	LIQUID AMOUNT	COOK TIME	COOKED BEANS
Aduki Beans	1 c.	4 c.	1½–2 hrs.	2½ c.
Black Eyed Peas	1 c.	3 c.	1 hr.	2½ c.
Lentils	1 c.	2½ c.	1 hr.	3 c.
Split Peas	1 c.	2 c.	45 min.	2¼ c.
Small Limas	1 c.	2½ c.	1½ hr.	2¼ c.

SOAKED BEANS	DRY BEANS	LIQUID AMOUNT	SOAK TIME	COOK TIME	COOKED BEANS
Black Beans	1 c.	3½ c.	3 hrs.	1½ hrs.	2¾ c.
Chick Peas	1 c.	4 c.	overnight	3 hrs.	2½ c.
Great Northern	1 c.	2 c.	3 hrs.	1 hr. 15 min.	2 c.
Kidney Beans	1 c.	2 c.	3 hrs.	1½ hrs.	2 c.
Large Limas	1 c.	2½ c.	3 hrs.	1 hr. 15 min.	2¼ c.
Marrow Beans	1 c.	2 c.	3 hrs.	2 ½ hrs.	2 c.
Navy Beans	1 c.	3¼ c.	3 hrs.	1 hr. 15 min.	2½ c.
Pea Beans	1 c.	3¼ c.	3 hrs.	1 hr. 15 min.	2½ c.
Pinto Beans	1 c.	3½ c.	3 hrs.	2½ hrs.	2 c.
Red Beans	1 c.	3 c.	3 hrs.	3 hrs.	2 c.
Soy Beans	1 c.	4 c.	overnight	3 hrs.	3 c.

Reading This Chart

The list of beans is divided into those that need to be soaked, and those that do not need to be soaked.

For the unsoaked beans: Bring the required amount of water and beans close to the boil. Turn the heat down to the lowest possible setting, and cook for the time indicated.

For the soaked beans: Soak them for the time indicated. Drain and rinse. Then bring the soaked beans and fresh liquid close to a boil, turn the heat down to the lowest possible setting and cook for the time indicated.

BEAN RECIPES

HUMMUS (GARBANZO OR CHICK PEA DIP)

2 c. cooked chick peas
5 Tbl. tahini (¼ c. + 1 Tbl.)
¼ c. lemon juice
2 tsp. soy sauce
1½ tsp. olive oil
½ tsp. cumin (optional)

1 Tbl. minced parsley
2 cloves garlic, minced (about 1 tsp.)
About 2 Tbl. chick pea cook water, or enough so that the dip is not too thick.

Method for cooking chick peas:

1 c. dry beans = 2 to 2¾ c. cooked

Soak 1 c. dry beans in 4 c. water for 2–3 hours. To help get rid of the carbohydrate in the bean that causes gas, replace the soak water with fresh water after each hour.

Bring the beans to a boil in fresh water twice the volume of the beans. Cook on the lowest possible simmer for 2 to 3 hours, or until the beans are tender. You may need to add more water after 1 hour of simmering. Be sure that you always have enough water so that the beans do not burn.

To make the dip:

Put 2 cups of the cooked beans, plus all other ingredients listed above (tahini, lemon juice, soy sauce, olive oil, etc.) in a blender. Blend completely. Add more chick pea cooking water, if the dip is too thick.

Serve with whole grain pita bread or crackers, as a dip for raw vegetables, or as a sandwich spread.

LENTIL WALNUT BURGERS *(Makes 4 patties)*

⅓ c. dry lentils
¼ c. chopped onion
3 Tbl. chopped parsley
⅓ c. rye bread crumbs
⅓ c. chopped walnuts

½ to 1 tsp. thyme (1 tsp. is
  tasty if you like thyme.)
1 egg
2 tsp. olive oil
½ tsp. soy sauce

Put the dry lentils in a pot with one cup of water. Bring the water close to the boil, then turn it down to the lowest possible simmer. Let cook till soft—about ½ hour.

Meanwhile, chop the onion, parsley, and walnuts, and prepare the bread crumbs.

Sauté the onion in the oil on a low heat.

In a large bowl, mix together the walnut pieces, bread crumbs and thyme.

When the lentils are done, drain them, then put them in a blender with the sautéed onion, the soy sauce, egg and parsley. Blend till broken down, but not liquid.

Pour the lentil mixture into the bowl of the dry mixture. Mix them together.

Form about 4 patties and put them on a lightly greased baking sheet.

Bake at 350° for 20 minutes.

Delicious hot or cold as is, with tomato sauce, or on a whole grain English muffin with sugar-free ketchup.

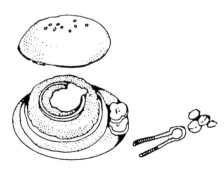

WILD RICE & BEAN LOAF WITH MUSHROOM GRAVY

Loaf:

3 eggs or 2 eggs and 2 egg whites	1 medium onion, chopped
3 c. cooked navy beans	1 clove garlic, minced
2 c. cooked wild rice	1¼ c. chopped mushrooms
2 tsp. olive oil	⅔ c. chopped celery
	optional: 1 tsp. vegetable salt

Beat the eggs in a large bowl.

Add the beans and rice. Stir, then transfer to a blender. Blend briefly so that you have mostly "mush," with some beans and rice left unmashed. Put the mixture back in the bowl.

Sauté the onion, garlic, mushrooms and celery in the oil. Add it to the bean/rice mixture. (Also add the vegetable salt, if you like.) Mix well.

Pour into a lightly greased baking pan. Bake at 350° 30 to 40 minutes.

Top with gravy. You can use the Super Sauce gravy with ginger (p. 194), or the Super Sauce with garlic and cumin. Or, try the following mushroom gravy:

Mushroom Gravy (Makes 1⅓ c.)

1 Tbl. butter/olive oil combination	1 c. water
⅓ c. chopped onion	1 Tbl. kuzu
1 c. chopped mushrooms	¼ tsp. soy sauce

Sauté the onion and mushroom in the butter. In the blender, blend the water, kuzu and soy sauce. Add the sautéed onion and mushroom. Blend briefly again, then transfer back to the sauté pan and simmer on a low heat, stirring constantly till thick.

BEAN SALAD WITH MUSTARD DRESSING

2 c. cooked great northern beans

1 c. cooked green spinach macaroni

⅔ c. sliced carrot (approximately 1 large carrot), raw or lightly steamed

2 stalks celery, chopped in small pieces

1½ c. broccoli flowerettes, raw or lightly steamed

¼ c. chopped parsley

¾ c. sliced mushrooms

Combine the above ingredients. Mix with the following dressing:

Mustard Dressing   Makes ½ c.

Mix or blend well:

2 Tbl. apple cider vinegar

2 Tbl. mustard

2 Tbl. tahini

2 to 3 Tbl. water

½ tsp. tarragon

For Chicken Salad:

This recipe also makes a great chicken salad. Use cooked diced chicken in place of cooked beans.

TOFU

For some people, tofu, or "soy bean curd," is a new and exotic food. However, because of its bland taste, it is extremely versatile. Try incorporating it into your diet gradually, adding it to sauces, soups, noodle dishes, grain dishes, or desserts. Or, try the following simple recipes.

SCRAMBLED TOFU

16 oz. firm tofu, cut in small cubes
¼ c. chopped fresh parsley
1⅓ c. sliced mushrooms (about 8 large mushrooms)
⅓ c. chopped red pepper
⅓ c. chopped scallions (2 medium sized)
1½ Tbl. olive oil
1 tsp. soy sauce
¼ tsp. ground marjoram
¼ tsp. turmeric

Sauté the scallions and mushrooms on a low heat in a large skillet. Add the remaining ingredients. Scramble gently till warm and well mixed (3 to 4 minutes).

Add a pinch of cayenne pepper.

BROILED TOFU

Mix your favorite vegetable broth powder, soy sauce, water, minced garlic and ground ginger. Slice the tofu thin and dip in the broth mixture. Marinate 1 hour or more. Place the tofu on a flat pan and put the pan under the broiler. Broil till fairly dry (about 10 minutes on a side).

Snacks & Desserts

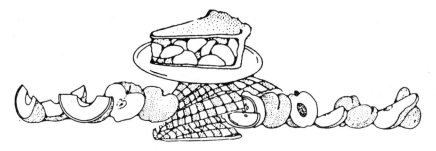

For muffins and dessert breads, such as Millet Banana Bread, Zucchini Bread and Gingerbread, see Breads and Muffins.

Note that in this section I have used certain ingredients that may not be recommended for over-all health, such as butter, eggs and nuts and seeds. An occasional dessert containing these ingredients should be fine, especially as part of a transition diet. In addition certain nuts and seeds, especially almonds and walnuts, are in the beneficial family of fats.

RECIPES

SUNNY SALTY SNACK (*Makes 2½ c.*)

Nuts and seeds are more nutritious raw, but this is a delicious transition snack. It is a perfect holiday or house-warming gift, packaged in an attractive jar.

1 c. walnuts	¼ tsp. cayenne pepper
¼ c. soy sauce	¼ tsp. ground celery seeds
1½ Tbl. oil	1 c. sunflower seeds
⅛ tsp. paprika	½ c. pumpkin seeds

Put the walnuts in a shallow pan. Cover with the soy sauce. Soak overnight.

The next day, drain the soy sauce into a small bowl, leaving the walnuts in the pan.

Mix into the soy sauce the oil, cayenne, paprika and ground celery seeds. Add the sunflower seeds and mix until they are thoroughly coated with the mixture.

Add the coated sunflower seeds to the soaked walnuts in the shallow pan. Bake in a preheated oven at 350° for 10 minutes.

Let cook, then mix the baked walnuts and sunflower seeds with the pumpkin seeds.

SNACKS TO GO

Mix any of the following to munch any time, remembering that nuts and seeds are high in calories, and can contribute to weight gain.

- almonds
- walnuts
- shredded coconut
- soaked dried fruit

- sunflower seeds
- pumpkin seeds
- dulse

QUICK CANDIES (*Makes 15 quarter sized, rich tasting candies*)

3 Tbl. ground almonds (or more, if you plan to roll the candies in almond meal)

2 Tbl. pure carob powder

2 Tbl. tahini

4 tsp. honey, barley malt or rice bran syrup

1 tsp. vanilla extract

Mix the ground almonds and carob powder. Add the tahini, honey, vanilla and any flavoring variations listed below, depending on which taste you prefer. Mix well. Form into small candies. Pat with ground almonds or sesame seeds. Refrigerate.

Note: Any time you have left over almond meal, prepare a glass of almond milk to enjoy with your candies.

Variations:

For carob mint kisses, add 2 drops peppermint oil.
For carob orange candies, add ¼ tsp. orange extract.
For sesame marzipan, add 2 Tbl. shredded coconut and
    ½ tsp almond extract.

SWEET TREATS

Delicious candies can be made by mixing any of the following ingredients:

- ground or whole nuts and seeds

- rehydrated dried fruit

- sprouts

- shredded coconut

- nut butter such as almond or tahini

- unsweetened carob powder

- powdered coffee substitute

- vanilla, orange or almond extract

- peppermint, spearmint or wintergreen oil

- pure fruit juice or apple cider

- honey, maple syrup, molasses, barley malt or rice bran syrup

CAROB GRAHAM CRACKERS

Put either of the following combinations of ingredients in a Cuisinart or strong blender and blend to a thick paste. Add spring water if necessary:

1 handful almonds	2 Tbl. honey
2 Tbl. unsweetened carob powder	2 Tbl. butter

or

1 handful almonds	2 tsp. honey
1 Tbl. tahini	⅛ tsp. vanilla extract
2 black mission figs	
2 Tbl. unsweetened carob powder	

Spread on or between honey graham crackers, rye or wheat crackers.

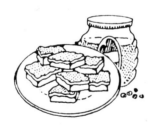

CAROB BROWNIES

(Don't expect chocolate brownies. Do expect delicious carob brownies!)

Dry Ingredients:

½ c. oat flour or ¾ c. rye flour   ½ c. filbert flour (approximately
½ c. carob powder   ⅓ c. filbert nuts ground fine)
1 tsp. baking soda   ¾ c. chopped pecans or walnuts

Note: If you can't find filberts, use almonds, or an additional ⅓ c. flour. The filberts contribute to a "chocolate" taste, but the brownies will be good without them. Oat flour has a more moist and chewy texture than rye flour.

Wet ingredients:

2 eggs, beaten or 1 egg plus 2   1 Tbl. molasses
  egg whites   2 tsp. vanilla extract
¾ c. honey   ½ c. melted butter (1 stick)

Preheat the oven to 350°.

Sift together the oat or rye flour, the carob powder and the baking soda. Stir in the filbert flour and the chopped nuts.

In another bowl, mix the wet ingredients, then add them to the dry. Stir till well mixed.

Pour the batter into a lightly greased pan. Use a 9" x 13" pan for a chewy texture, or a 9" x 9" pan for a cake texture.

Bake at 350° for 25 to 30 minutes.

Remove from the oven while it is still somewhat moist in the center. It will become more firm and dry as it cools and will fall slightly. Let cool before eating.

CAROB CHIP COOKIES (*Makes about 2 dozen cookies*)

5 Tbl. butter
1 Tbl. molasses
½ c. honey
½ tsp. vanilla extract
1 c. whole wheat pastry or
   brown rice flour

½ tsp. baking soda
1 egg
½ c. chopped walnuts
½ c. unsweetened carob chips

Preheat the oven to 375°.

Cream together the butter, honey and molasses.

In a separate bowl, mix the flour and baking soda.

Add the vanilla and egg to the butter mixture. Mix well, then add the flour and baking soda.

Mix well. Add the chopped walnuts and carob chips. Mix.

Refrigerate the dough 1 hour.

Lightly grease a baking sheet.

Drop the dough mixture in tablespoon-sized circles, about 1 inch apart, onto the baking sheet.

Bake at 375° for 8–10 minutes.

OATMEAL COOKIES (*Makes 40 cookies*)

Preheat the oven to 350°.

Wet ingredients:

2 eggs, beaten
½ c. melted butter
½ c. honey or ⅓ c. barley malt

1 tsp. blackstrap molasses
½ tsp. vanilla extract

Dry ingredients:

2 c. rolled oats
½ c. ground rolled oats
¼ tsp. baking soda

½ tsp. cinnamon
¾ c. raisins
optional: ¾ c. chopped nuts

Beat the eggs, then add the other wet ingredients. Stir till well mixed.

In a large bowl, combine the dry ingredients. Add the wet ingredients to the dry. Stir till well mixed.

Drop the cookie batter onto a lightly greased cookie sheet by level tablespoons. You may need to mold them a tiny bit, if the dough doesn't hold together well.

Bake at 350° for 12–15 minutes.

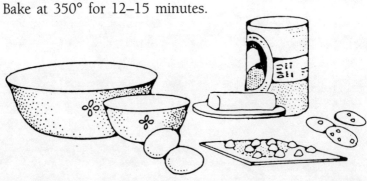

CARROT CAKE

Preheat the oven to 350°.

For this recipe, use a lightly greased bundt pan, or two 9" spring form layer pans, if you wish to layer the cake. The bundt pan makes a very pretty (and delicious) cake that is great for tea time. If you use the layer pans, a lemon frosting is delicious.

Wet ingredients:

3 eggs or 2 eggs + 2 egg whites	½ c. plain yogurt
	½ c. melted butter
¾ c. honey	2 c. grated carrots

Dry ingredients:

2 c. whole wheat pastry flour	(For a spicy cake, add ½ tsp. allspice)
1 tsp. baking soda	
1¼ tsp. cinnamon	

In a medium bowl, beat the eggs, then add the other wet ingredients. Stir till well mixed.

In a large bowl, combine the dry ingredients, stirring with a wire whisk.

Add the wet ingredients to the dry, stirring till well-mixed.

Pour the batter into the greased bundt pan or the layer pans.

Bake at 350° for 45 to 50 minutes.

ALMOND TORTE—*flour free (Makes two 9" layers)*

6 eggs, separated
½ c. honey
2 tsp. vanilla extract
¼ tsp. almond extract
2½ Tbl. lemon juice and 1½ Tbl. lemon peel (1 lemon)

¼ c. cooked baking potato (about 3 oz. potato, skinned, diced, simmered and cooled in cold water to room temperature)
2 c. ground unblanched almonds (1½ c. unground. Grind ⅓ c. at a time)

Preheat the oven to 350°.

Prepare two 9" cake pans: Grease the bottoms, but not the sides of the pans. Line the bottoms with brown paper or parchment paper, cut to fit. Don't grease the paper.

In a large bowl, beat the egg yolks with an electric mixer until they are thick and lemon-colored (about 6 minutes). Add the honey, a small amount at a time, beating another 15 minutes. Add the lemon peel, juice, and extracts, then the ¼ c. potato, and mix again.

Add the ground almonds, a small amount at a time, mixing them in very well.

In a separate large bowl, beat the egg whites with an electric mixer until the whites form soft peaks, but are not dry.

Gently fold the whites into the batter.

Bake 40 to 50 minutes at 350°.

Let the cake cool in the pan on a wire rack before removing. (It will fall slightly.) Then, carefully loosen the torte from the sides with a knife, and remove. Let cool before serving, or adding icing.

Serve as is, or with carob mint sauce (p. 272), kefir cheese, fresh fruit, lemon icing, carob icing, or carob-orange icing. If you use carob orange icing, I don't recommend layering it, as the icing is very rich.

BASIC VANILLA CAKE

Makes two 9" layers.
Preheat the oven to 350°.

½ c. honey	1⅓ c. whole wheat pastry flour
6 large eggs	6 Tbl. melted butter
1¼ tsp. vanilla extract	

Lightly grease two 9" layer pans, and dust them with flour.

Melt the butter, and set it aside.

The secret to this cake is mixing the eggs with an electric beater until they are high and thick. This works best if the eggs, mixing bowl and beaters are slightly warm. Simmer some water in the bottom half of a large double boiler, or any large pot. Place over the pot (but not in the water) the top of the double boiler, or any large pan or stainless steel mixing bowl.

Pour the honey into the pot or mixing bowl, then add the eggs and vanilla. Dip the electric beaters into the simmering water to warm them.

With the electric mixer at medium speed, beat the honey and eggs until the mixture is very thick and high, approximately 12 to 15 minutes.

With a rubber spatula, gently fold in the flour, thoroughly mixing a small amount at a time. Then, slowly add the melted butter, thoroughly folding it in until well mixed.

Pour the batter into the two cake pans, and bake at 350° for 30–40 minutes, or until the cake is golden brown and pulls away from the sides of the pan. Let cool on a wire rack.

Variations:

Add the grated rind of 2 small lemons. or in place of the vanilla extract, use 1 tsp. almond extract or 2 Tbl. rum.

You could also make cupcakes out of this batter. Fill the muffin tins ⅓ full, and bake in a preheated oven at 375° for 20–25 minutes. Top with carob or lemon icing.

CAKE TOPPING IDEAS

Top each layer with carob, lemon, almond or orange icing.

Sprinkle the top with chopped or sliced nuts; or,

Decorate with fresh strawberries or flowers. If you like, put a dollop of plain yogurt or whipped cream or kefir cheese under each strawberry.

Cakes are also delicious with fresh fruit in between the layers, such as mashed raspberries.

Or, instead of using a frosting, pour carob mint sauce (p. 272) over a one-layer cake.

ICINGS

Note: Eva's Carob Frosting and the Lemon Frosting tend to melt a bit. It sometimes helps to put the frostings in the refrigerator for about 45 minutes to set and to put them on a cooled cake.

It may also help to refrigerate the cake after you have put the icing on, but before you have smoothed the icing out on the top and sides. It is worth the trouble!

If the carob frosting is difficult to spread, try dipping a knife in a cup of hot water, shaking off the excess water, and spreading the frosting with the hot knife.

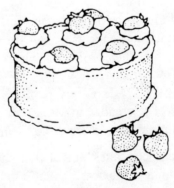

ICING RECIPES

Eva's Carob Frosting (*Enough for two 9" layers.*)

1 c. honey	2 Tbl. vanilla extract
1 c. softened butter	1½ c. unsweetened carob powder

Stir the ingredients with a spoon till the carob is mixed in. (Otherwise, when you turn on the mixer, you may get a surprise dusting.) Beat the ingredients with a mixer until it is a frosting consistency.

Alternate: For a delicious carob/orange frosting, add 2 tsp. pure orange extract.

Lemon Frosting:

⅓ c. honey	¼ c. ground almonds
2 Tbl. sweet butter	
Grated peel from 1 organic	
lemon (approximately 2 Tbl.)	

Melt the butter on a low heat in a small sauce pan. Meanwhile, grind the almonds in a blender or food processor. Add the melted butter, honey and lemon peel and blend till well mixed.

ALMOND FROSTING:

¼ c. honey

3 Tbl. butter, softened

⅔ c. finely ground almonds

⅓ c. unsweetened carob powder

4 Tbl. cream, or 3 Tbl. kefir cheese

½ tsp. almond extract

In a medium mixing bowl, cream the honey and butter. Add the ground almonds and carob powder and mix well. Add the cream and almond extract and beat until smooth.

RAW FRUIT PIES

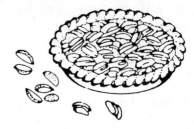

CRUST:

¾ lb. soft dates, pitted and chopped

2 c. ground walnuts

Knead the crust ingredients together. Press into a 10" pie plate. Refrigerate overnight to help it to harden. Fill with the "Mixed Fruit Filling."

FILLING: MIXED DRIED FRUITS

Soak 1 cup of a mixture of dried fruit (such as apricots, prunes, pears and raisins) in the following liquid:

1–2 c. water, or enough water so that there is about ½ inch above the fruit.

juice of ½ large lemon or 1 small lemon
½ tsp. cinnamon

In the morning, pour off or strain the juice. (Save for a sauce.) Add more lemon juice and cinnamon, if you like. Put the dried fruit mixture into the pie crust. Serve as is, or chill it first.

Optional:

Sprinkle with shredded coconut.

APPLE FILLING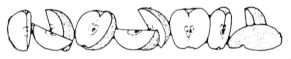

Prepare the Raw Fruit Pie Crust, then fill with a combination of fresh apples and raisins which have been soaked overnight in lemon juice and cinnamon.

RAW APPLESAUCE

2 apples, cored and sliced in
   chunks
1 Tbl. raisins

½ tsp. cinnamon
2 Tbl. apple cider or apple
   juice

Optional Additions:

½ banana
   dates or currants in place of
   raisins

pinch of cloves

Put the apples and the juice in the blender and blend well. While blending, add the raisins and spices (and banana). Add more liquid and cinnamon, if necessary.

Serve at room temperature, or slightly warm.

DRIED FRUIT COMPOTE

Use one or more of any of the following unsulfured dried fruits:

apricots	pears	prunes	peaches
apples	figs	raisins	

Soak overnight in a combination of water, lemon juice and cinnamon. Use enough liquid so that there is about ½ inch surplus liquid over the surface of the fruit. The fruit will absorb much of the liquid and will expand. Don't cook.

Before serving, add more lemon juice and/or cinnamon to taste.

Easy Apple Tarts

Jelled Filling (Makes 2 cups):

1 apple, coarsely chopped	2½ Tbl. grated lemon peel
1½ c. apple juice	½ tsp. ground cinnamon
2 Tbl. pure pectin	

Blend briefly in a blender so that it is mixed, but you still have some apple chunks. Then add and stir:

⅓ c. raisins

Let sit in the refrigerator 2–4 hours, or until jelled.

Note that if you just want a jello, you can eat this as is without a crust. Put it in individual glass bowls or champagne glasses. Sprinkle the top with grated coconut or grated lemon peel. You can also add granola to the jello for a crunchy texture.

Crust:

1 c. ground granola. Grind it so that you still have some small chunks left.	6 Tbl. soft butter

Preheat the oven to 350°.

Mix the ground granola and soft butter by rubbing them in your hands. When they stick together, line the bottom of 6 individual baking cups with about ¼" of the mixture. Bake at 350° for 10 minutes. Remove the cups from the oven and let cool at least 10 minutes.

Fill the cups with the jelled mixture. Sprinkle with grated lemon peel.

PINEAPPLE-TOFU CUSTARD

Blend drained tofu and drained pineapple to taste. Add honey and vanilla extract to taste.

POPCORN, PLUS

Popcorn can be a wonderful and nutritious snack. It becomes un-healthy by cooking it in oils which are too hot, which then become toxic, or by covering it with rancid oils. Popcorn is best made by using a non-aluminum screen or basket type popper, popping it dry over a hot stove or flame, or by using a non-aluminum air-type popper.

After popping, add any of the following in any combinations:

- melted butter
- soy sauce
- nutritional yeast
- cinnamon
- vegetable salt
- dried basil, garlic or onion powder

- melted butter + oil
- garlic, or garlic oil
- grated Parmesan cheese
- cayenne pepper
- powdered kelp or dulse

To make garlic oil, blenderize minced garlic with a good raw olive oil.

FROZEN FRUIT "LICK STICKS"

FROZEN BANANAS

Peel and freeze a banana, then eat as is, or make a Carob Banana.

Carob Banana:

For 2–3 bananas, sliced in halves or thirds:

¼ c. unsweetened carob powder   2 Tbl. water

Optional: vanilla or almond extract to taste

Mix the above ingredients until a thick paste. Roll the banana slices in the paste, then in ½ c. chopped nuts and/or shredded coconut Put the coated banana sticks in the freezer till hard.

FROZEN FRUIT STICKS

Purchase popsicle sticks and molds, or use small cans from frozen concentrated fruit juice. Fill the molds or cans with any of the following:

- pure juice: grape, apple, orange, pineapple, papaya, mango
- peppermint tea with lemon juice and honey
- sugar-free yogurt
- layers of yogurt and fruit juice
- frozen fruit ice cream
- sliced fresh fruit blended with water

Put the stick in the mold, then put the mold in the freezer till solid.

FRESH FRUIT ICE CREAM

BANANA ICE CREAM

Peel 3 ripe bananas, cut them in chunks, and put them in the freezer on a plate or wax paper. Freeze until hard, or nearly hard.

Put the chunks, a few at a time, into a blender, food processor or Champion juicer. If using a blender, you will occasionally need to stop the blender and use a rubber spatula to push the pieces down. If your blender is not too powerful, the chunks may bounce around at first. Be patient. Soon they will "catch" and become ice cream consistency. Sometimes it helps to add some unfrozen banana to the blender.

ICE CREAM TOPPINGS

- raisins or other rehydrated dried fruit
- chopped nuts
- fresh fruit, such as peaches, blueberries, strawberries, raspberries
- carob syrup
- shredded coconut

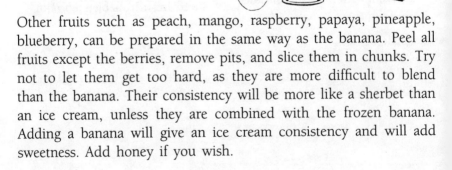

FRESH FRUIT SHERBET

Other fruits such as peach, mango, raspberry, papaya, pineapple, blueberry, can be prepared in the same way as the banana. Peel all fruits except the berries, remove pits, and slice them in chunks. Try not to let them get too hard, as they are more difficult to blend than the banana. Their consistency will be more like a sherbet than an ice cream, unless they are combined with the frozen banana. Adding a banana will give an ice cream consistency and will add sweetness. Add honey if you wish.

Fruity Banana

Freeze the banana as per the banana ice cream recipe. Freeze any other fruits per the sherbet recipe, or purchase unsweetened pure frozen fruit.

Blend together an equal amount of frozen banana and any other frozen fruit. Some delicious combinations are as follows:

- banana + peach
- banana + papaya
- banana + mango
- banana + strawberries
- banana + raspberries
- banana + pineapple

Banana Split

Slice unfrozen bananas and put them in a bowl. Top with fresh fruit ice cream of your choice, then with any ice cream toppings.

Quick Dessert with Carob Mint or Mocha Sauce

Pour carob mint, mocha, orange or almond sauce over any of the following:

- Fresh strawberries, or any other fresh fruit (kiwis, papaya, mango, peaches, pears, bananas, blueberries, apples, or any combination)
- Poached fruit, such as poached pear
- Fresh fruit ice cream or sherbet
- Honey vanilla, or honey carob ice cream, or any other sugar-free, pure ice cream
- One layer cake, such as almond torte

BASIC CAROB SAUCE: (*Makes 1 cup*)

Blend in a blender:

½ c. hot water
½ c. honey
⅓ c. tahini
1 Tbl. vanilla extract
¾ c. unsweetened carob powder

Note that this sauce thickens in the refrigerator. You may need to add about ¼ c. more water, in that case.

Variations:

For a carob mint sauce, add 2 drops peppermint oil. (Use a dropper.)

For a mocha sauce, add grain coffee substitute, such as Pero or Cafix to taste.

For a carob orange sauce, add 1 tsp. orange extract.

Use your own imagination, mixing the different extracts with mocha and carob, and adding the sauce to other favorite desserts.

SECTION IV

APPENDIX

Natural Food Kitchen Hints

CLEANING VEGETABLES

Add to a sinkful of water 1 tsp. apple cider vinegar, Clorox, or wheatgrass juice. Soak fruits and vegetables (except onions) in their skins in the water for about 5 minutes. Drain, rinse, and dry. This helps cut the residue of pesticides that may remain on the skin of the vegetable or fruit.

KEEPING FOODS FRESH

GREENS

- Greens will keep well if wrapped in paper towels or a dish towel, then stored in a plastic bag in the refrigerator.
- Or, store your vegetables in the refrigerator vegetable bin which has been lined with paper towels or napkins. You can also put dry sponges in the vegetable bin. Any of these methods helps absorb excess moisture which rots the greens.
- To perk up wilted greens, pick off the brown edges, then sprinkle the greens with cool water. Wrap them in a cloth

or paper towel and refrigerate at least one hour. Or, dip the greens in cool water to which has been added 1 tsp. lemon juice or apple cider vinegar or a few slices of raw potato. Then wrap and refrigerate.

- If you need wet greens dried quickly, put them in a pillow case and spin-dry in the washing machine.
- Keep parsley, watercress, and any fresh herbs refrigerated in a wide-mouthed glass jar with a tight lid.
- Parsley can be frozen, or can be dried by placing it on a cookie sheet in the oven with the pilot light for a few days. Store it in a glass jar after it is completely dried.

TOFU

- Keep tofu refrigerated in a container of water, making sure the water covers the tofu. Change the water daily, if possible.

GRAINS, NUTS & SEEDS, FLOUR & OIL

- Oil-based foods should be kept in the refrigerator and, whenever possible, in the freezer (particularly when there is a long storage time). This helps prevent rancidity (particularly when kept in the freezer) and bug infestation. Keeping them in glass jars is preferable since paper or cellophane bags can become soggy from melting ice.

If you buy any of these foods in bulk, keep the majority of it in the freezer, and keep smaller quantities easily available in the refrigerator.

BREADS

- Put a stalk of celery or ½ apple in a bread box with the bread.
- To thaw frozen bread quickly, heat it in the oven in a brown paper bag for about 5 minutes at 325°.
- To freshen dried bread, wrap it in a damp towel, refrigerate it for 24 hours, then remove the towel and heat the bread in the oven for a few minutes.

EGGS

- To help prevent eggs from picking up bacteria, leave them in their cartons in the refrigerator rather than storing them in the egg slots on the refrigerator door. The inside of the refrigerator is colder than the temperatures on the refrigerator door (cold inhibits the bacteria) and the egg cartons are less likely to be contaminated with bacteria than the refrigerator door. Store the eggs with the large end up, the tapered end down. (This helps keep the yolk away from the egg's natural air pocket, a potential breeding ground for bacteria. The yolk is more perishable than the white.) Storing eggs in the original carton will also help prevent them from picking up odors from the refrigerator.
- When separating whites from yolks, use an egg separator rather than the shell.
- When using raw eggs in a recipe such as mayonnaise, two tablespoons of vinegar or lemon juice to one cup of oil will inhibit the growth of bacteria.
- To determine the freshness of an egg, put it in a bowl of cold water. If it sinks and lies on its side, it's fresh; if it sinks but stands partially or fully erect, it's not fresh, but still edible; if it floats to the top, it's rotten.

MISCELLANEOUS KITCHEN HINTS

TO LIQUEFY CRYSTALLIZED HONEY:

- Put the honey jar in a pot of hot water and let it stand until the honey is melted.

TO MEASURE HONEY:

- Lightly oil a measuring cup, or measure the oil before the honey in your recipe. The honey will easily slide out of an oiled measuring cup.

TO QUICKEN THE RIPENING PROCESS:

- Bury avocados in a bowl full of flour.
- Put green bananas and green tomatoes in a wet towel, then in a brown paper bag.

WHEN YOU NEED JUST A LITTLE LEMON JUICE:

- Poke a hole in the lemon, then squeeze.
- Or, slice a small piece off the end of the lemon and use that. Put the rest of the lemon in saran wrap.

STORING JARS AND LIDS:

• To keep the right lid with the right jar without closing the jar (which can encourage the growth of bacteria in the jar): Hold the lid to the side of the jar with a rubber band.

EGG HINTS:

• *How to tell if your egg is raw or cooked:* Spin the egg on its side on a flat surface. If it wobbles, it is raw; if it rotates smoothly, it is hard cooked. (In an uncooked egg the yolk will move around, changing the egg's center of gravity.)
• *Peeling a hard boiled egg:* Start at the larger end, or hold it under cold water.
• *To slice a hard boiled egg without it crumbling:* Refrigerate it first for 15 minutes.
• *Safe microwaving:* Always pierce the yolk of an egg before cooking; otherwise it can explode and cause serious burns.

HINTS FOR CLEANING UTENSILS

It is helpful in setting up your kitchen to keep the utensils most often used near your work space and, if possible, near the sink. For example, have a hanging rack where small utensils such as measuring spoons and cup, grater, wire whisk, etc, can drip dry.

Try to wash utensils and equipment as soon as possible after use, so that dried out food does not stick to them. If this is not convenient, put them in a sink or dish pan full of hot water until you can wash them thoroughly. Or, fill your used pots and pans and measuring cup with hot water and put the utensils in them until future washing.

Be sure to leave all blenders and juicers uncovered after washing, to air them out and help prevent the growth of bacteria.

BLENDER:

- If it is not possible to scrub your blender right away, fill it with water and clean it later.
- Or, fill the blender half way with water and add a drop of detergent. Blend, covered, for a few seconds. Rinse and let drain dry.

GARLIC PRESS:

- Put the garlic press in hot water right away after use, as it is difficult to remove dried pieces of garlic. If necessary, use a toothpick to remove the garlic pieces.

GRATER:

- Use an old toothbrush to remove lemon peel, onion, cheese, etc. from your grater.

• Before using the grater, rub it with olive oil to prevent food from sticking to it.

CUTTING BOARD:

• To remove onion or garlic smell, cut a lemon or lime and rub the board with the cut end of the fruit.

COMMON FOOD ADDITIVES

This list, comprising the additives most commonly listed on packaged foods, is to assist you in reading labels.

NAME	FUNCTION	USED IN	LEVEL OF TOXICITY
Acesulfame-K (Sunette or Sweet One)	Artificial sweetener	Soft drinks and baked goods	Toxic. Causes cancer in laboratory animals.
Agar (A carbohydrate extracted from seaweed)	Prevent icing from drying out. Gelling ingredient.	Cup cakes	Non-toxic
Artificial Color and Artificial Flavor	Used to entice consumer to buy the product	Commercially packaged cereals, candy, jams, ice cream, cheese, baked goods, butter, dessert powder, fruit skins (such as lemon and orange), packaged sausage, soft drinks.	No nutritive value. Disguises lack of nutritious ingredients and age. Color: Coal tar dyes are suspected carcinogens. Tests have shown high levels of toxicity in some of the dyes. Flavor: Little testing has been done.
Aspartame (Nutra Sweet or Equal)	Artificial sweetener	Soft drinks and baked goods	Toxic. May cause mental retardation in babies with a genetic disease called phenylketonuria and may cause dizziness, headaches, epileptic-like seizures and menstrual problems in sensitive individuals.
Benzoic Acid	Flavor preservative and anti-mold ingredient	Jams, jellies, beverages, candies. Also used in ice for cooling fish.	Toxic. Tests on humans showed irritation to eyes, skin and mucous membranes. Tests on rats resulted in retarded growth, brain damage and possibly cancer.
Brominated Vegetable Oil	Used to make the oils look cloudy, which gives the appearance of thickness	Oils	Insufficient testing. Some studies have shown harmful effects to animal's heart, kidneys, liver, thyroid and testicles.

Additive	Purpose	Found In	Toxicity
BHA (Butylated Hydroxyanisole) and BHT (Butylated Hydroxytoluene)	Anti-oxidants; that is, prevents polyunsaturated oils from oxidizing and becoming rancid.	Cake mixes, cereals, breads, crackers, dry soups, pork, instant teas, vegetable oils, steak sauces	Toxic. Tests done on rats showed that their cholesterol levels rose, hair fell out, and they were born without eyes.
Caffeine	Stimulant	Coffee, soft drinks, chocolate and most non-herbal teas	May cause nervousness, nausea, insomnia. May also promote breast lumps and interfere with reproduction and fetal development.
Calcium Disodium EDTA (Ethylenediamine tetraacetate)	Helps promote and retain color, flavor and texture.	Soft drinks, canned vegetables, sauces, spreads, dressings	Toxic. Tests on humans resulted in kidney damage, vitamin and mineral imbalance, gastrointestinal distress and muscle cramps.
Caramel	For flavor and color	Instant teas, bread, soft drinks, candies	Being tested by FDA. Possibly toxic.
Carrageenan, or "Irish Moss" (A seaweed extract)	Suspending agent, stabilizer, thickener, emulsifier, gelling ingredient	Chocolate drinks, soft drinks, fruit juices, alcohol, vinegar, milk products & cheese, frozen desserts, soups, sauces, dressings, canned meats, baked goods	Non toxic, although tests with large amounts showed ulcers in animals. Low dosages have been used for medicinal purposes.
Citric Acid	Anti-oxidant. Prevents spoilage and discoloration of food. Adds a tart flavor.	Jellos, juices	Safe.
Dextrose	Sweetener	Canned soups, dressings, many processed foods.	Toxic as any sugar.
Gums: Arabic, cellulose, ghatti, karaya, tragacanth, xanthan	Improve texture (as in ice cream), prevent sugar from crystallizing; stabilize foam in beer; hold flavor in drink mixes; thickener	Candy, beer, ice cream, powdered drink mixes, colas	Insufficient testing. May cause allergic reactions such as diarrhea or constipation.

NAME	FUNCTION	USED IN	LEVEL OF TOXICITY
Hydrolyzed Vegetable Protein (or protein hydrolysate)	Flavor enhancer	Many processed foods.	Toxic. Contains MSG (See MSG). Tests showed damage to brains of infant mice.
Modified Food Starch	Binder, filler, stabilizer; makes the food resistant to high temperature and helps prevent doughy, rough or watery textures.	Bread, baked goods, baby food, soups, sauces, pie fillings, prepared dinner products, frozen pizza, frozen fish, canned corn, dry roasted nuts.	Being tested. Nutritionally worthless, often replacing more nutritious ingredients. Tests on humans indicate that it is difficult to digest, and may raise blood cholesterol levels.
Mono- and Di-glycerides	Prevent oil from separating; make cakes and breads soft and keep them from becoming stale by preventing starch from crystallizing	Peanut butter, cup cakes, bread, margarine, broths, shortenings	Being tested by FDA. May cause birth defects, genetic changes, cancer.
MSG (monosodium glutamate)	Flavor enhancer and appetite stimulator	Soups, sauces, salad dressings, processed cheese, Chinese food, dry roasted nuts, canned meats, frankfurters, frozen pizza	Toxic. Can cause headaches and tightness of chest. Lab tests on mice revealed brain damage, damage to the retina of the eye, and injury to the mouse fetus.
"Natural Sweeteners"	To sweeten a product.		Chemically refined cane juice. A toxic sugar.
Oatrim	Fat substitute	Meat, cheese, baked goods, frozen desserts	Safe. Extracted from oats.
Olestra	Fat substitute	Not yet approved for use	Toxic. Has caused liver damage and tumors in laboratory animals.
Potassium Sorbate	Prevent growth of molds and fungi	Cheese, mayonnaise, soft drinks, wine, dried fruit, margarine, canned frosting	Safe. A combination of sorbic acid and potassium.
Propionates - Calcium or Sodium	To prevent the growth of mold and certain bacteria	Breads	In general, the propionates are harmless, although some studies indicate allergic reactions, with symptoms of headaches and gastrointestinal stress similar to a gall bladder attack.

Name	Purpose	Found in	Notes
Propyl Gallate	Preservative	Vegetable oils and shortenings, chewing gum, pickles	Still being tested. Possibly toxic. May cause liver damage, birth defects.
Propylene Glycol Alginate	Thickener, stabilizer, solvent	Soft drinks, jelly, mustard, potato chips, crackers, cream cheese, yogurt, ice cream, frozen desserts	Being investigated by FDA. Substances in this additive are used for anti-freeze, oils and waxes.
Red Dye 40	Food coloring to entice the consumer	Red pistachio nuts, chewing gum, candies, frankfurters	Toxic. May be cancer-causing and cause birth defects.
Saccharin	To sweeten in place of sugar, since it costs the manufacturer $1/20$th as much as sugar and is 300 to 500 times sweeter.	Soft drinks, colas, puddings, powder mixes	Still being tested. Probably a carcinogen (cancer causing substance)
Simplesse	Fat substitute	Ice cream, dips, spreads, salad dressings and mayonnaise	Safe. Made from natural egg or milk protein.
Sodium Erythorbate	Preservative	Many baked goods and beverages, bacon, frankfurters	Toxic. Banned in several countries. May cause genetic defects.
Sodium Nitrate and Sodium Nitrite	Prevent the growth of bacteria that causes botulism. Improve color in meat by causing the pigment to turn red.	Packaged meats (bologna, salami, ham, corned beef, pastrami, etc.) sausage, frozen pizzas, bacon	Disguises age and poor quality of meat. Nitrites can lead to the formation of nitrosamines, proven cancer-causing substances. Under certain conditions, nitrates will become nitrites.
Sulfur Dioxide	Preservative, anti-oxidant and anti-browning agent.	Wine, corn syrup, dried fruit, glaceed fruit, imitation jelly, maraschino cherries, potato peels	Toxic. Tests on humans showed symptoms of nausea, headaches, listlessness, anemia, increased uric acid, destruction of blood corpuscles, dizziness, cramps, wheezing, death.

HIDDEN SUGARS

The following chart shows approximately how many teaspoons of sugar are added to certain food items. In addition to these, sugar is added to breakfast cereals (Some have more sugar than grain!), and many other canned and processed foods. Read labels.

FOOD	AMT.	APPROX. # TSP. SUGAR	FOOD	AMT.	APPROX. # TSP. SUGAR
Beverages			Canned stewed fruit	½ c.	2
Soft Drinks	12 oz.	8–10	Jello	½ c.	4½
Cordials	¾ oz.	1½	Chocolate pudding	½ c.	4
Hi-Ball	6 oz.	2½	Date or fig pudding	½ c.	7
Whiskey sour	3 oz.	1½			
Sweet cider	1 c.	6	Plum pudding	½ c.	4
Sweetened canned fruit juice	½ c.	2	Rice pudding	½ c.	5
			Tapioca pudding	½ c.	3
Dairy Products			Banana pudding	½ c.	2
Ice cream	⅓ pt.	3½	*Cakes, Cookies & Pastries*		
Ice cream cone	1	3½			
Ice cream soda	1	5	Average cakes & pastry	4 oz.	4–6
Ice cream sundae	1	7	Iced chocolate cake	4 oz.	10
Sherbet	½ c.	6			
Malted milk shake	10 oz.	5	Iced cup cake	1	6
Candies			Strawberry shortcake	1 piece	4
Chocolate bar	2 oz.	8	Plain donut	1	3
Chocolate mint	1	2	Glazed donut	1	6
Fudge	1 oz.	4½	Hamburger bun	1	3
Gum drop	1	2	Unfrosted brownie	¾ oz.	3
Hard candy	4 oz.	20	Chocolate cookie	1	1½
Life savers	1	½	Fig newton	1	5
Peanut brittle	1 oz.	3½	Ginger snap	1	3
Chewing gum	1 stick	½	Macaroon	1	6
Misc. Desserts			Nut cookie	1	1½
Canned apricots: 4 halves & 1 Tbl. syrup		3½	Oatmeal cookie	1	2
			Sugar cookie	1	1½
Canned peaches: 2 halves & 1 Tbl. syrup		3½	Chocolate eclair	1	7
Canned fruit salad	½ c.	3½	Cream puff	1	2

FOOD	AMT.	APPROX. # TSP. SUGAR	FOOD	AMT.	APPROX. # TSP. SUGAR
Brown Betty	½ c.	3	Chocolate sauce	1 Tbl.	3½
Pies: apple, lemon,			Canned fruit syrup	2 Tbl.	2½
peach, apricot	1 piece	7			
berry, cherry.	1 piece	10	Actual sugar content of the following:		
Condiments					
Ketchup	1 Tbl.	1	Corn syrup	1 Tbl.	3
Apple or peach	1 Tbl.	1	Karo syrup	1 Tbl.	3
butter			Brown sugar	1 Tbl.	3
			Granulated sugar	1 Tbl.	3
Syrup, Sugars & Icings			Maple syrup	1 Tbl.	5
Chocolate or white	1 oz.	3½	Molasses	1 Tbl.	3½
icing			Honey	1 Tbl.	3

HIDDEN SALT

The following chart shows the sodium content in common and processed foods. Note the difference between fresh and canned vegetables.

Food	Food Amt.	Approx. MG. of Sodium	Food	Food Amt.	Approx. MG. of Sodium
Cakes, Cookies, Snacks			Low fat milk/ yogurt	1 c.	120
Cheese crackers	10	325	Buttermilk	1 c.	275
Ritz crackers	9	288	Cottage cheese,		
Corn chips	1 oz.	231	creamed	c.	180
Potato chips	10	200	unsalted	c.	30
Pretzels	10	1,008	Parmesan cheese	1 Tbl.	40
Pillsbury sugar cookies	3	210	American cheese	1 oz.	320
Hostess Twinkies	1	240	Cheddar, Muenster, Swiss cheese	1 oz.	220
Popcorn, salted	1 c.	180	Low fat cheese	1 oz.	200
Popcorn, unsalted	1 c.	1	*Pharmaceuticals*		
Sweet roll	4"	240			
Doughnut	1	160	Alka Seltzer	1 dose	521
McDonald's apple pie	1	414	Bromo Seltzer	1 dose	717
			Brioschi	1 dose	710
Peanut brittle	1 oz.	145	Miles Nervine	1 dose	544
Peanuts, salted	c.	275	Fleet's Enema	1 dose	300
Peanuts, unsalted	c.	2	Metamucil Instant Mix	1 dose	250
Breads & Cereals			Rolaids	1 dose	53
Oatmeal, salted	1 c.	520	*Soups, Beverages*		
Kellogg's All Bran	c.	370			
Rice Krispies	1 c.	280	Soup, homemade, salted	1 c.	500
Puffed wheat, puffed rice, shredded wheat	1 c.	1	commercial, canned	1 c.	760
Corn flakes	1 c.	165	Instant broth mix	1 packet	818
Bran flakes	c.	340	McDonald chocolate shake	1	240
Bread	1 slice	130			
Dairy Products			*Meats*		
Butter, Margarine,			Beef, Veal	3 oz.	75
salted	1 Tbl.	140	McDonald's Big Mac	1	1,510
unsalted	1 Tbl.	1			

FOOD	FOOD AMT.	APPROX. MG. OF SODIUM	FOOD	FOOD AMT.	APPROX. MG. OF SODIUM
Chef Boyardee Beefaroni	7.5 oz.	1,186	*Miscellaneous*		
Ham, cured	3 oz.	675	Jello, instant	c.	404
Ham, uncured	3 oz.	560	Peanut butter, processed	2 Tbl.	172
Bacon	1 slice	75	homemade, unsalted	2 Tbl.	36
Canned franks/ beans	8 oz.	958	Ice cream	1 c.	42
Lamb, pork, chicken	3 oz.	75	Green olive	1	155
Frozen fried chicken	1 dinner	1,152	Dill pickle	1 large	1,400
			Miso	1 Tbl.	500
Frankfurter	1	540	Soy sauce	1 Tbl.	1,300
Bologna	1 slice	390	Salt	1 tsp.	2,300
Canned tuna fish	3 oz.	430	Commercial dressing	1 Tbl.	200–300
Fresh fish (except shell)	3 oz.	75	McDonald's Egg McMuffin	1	914
Vegetables & Beans			Worcestershire sauce	1 Tbl.	315
Asparagus, fresh	6 spears	4	Frozen pizza	2 oz.	328
canned	6 spears	410	Commercial ketchup	1 Tbl.	200
Peas, fresh	3 oz.	2			
canned	3 oz.	236	Commercial mustard	1 Tbl.	212
Green Beans, fresh	1 c.	5	Processed baby food	3 oz.	293–510
canned	1 c.	925	Instant vanilla pudding	1 c.	840
Corn, fresh	1 c.	5			
canned	1 c.	500	French fries	medium serving	150
Dry beans, unsalted	c.	15	Spaghetti sauce	4 oz.	800
salted	c.	350			

QUICK PLANNED MENUS

These menus include quick recipes, and illustrate simple preparation techniques that are suggested in this book. Wait 1 to 1 ½ hours before dessert to aid digestion.

BREAKFAST	LUNCH	DINNER
Green drink Oatmeal with nut milk Special calcium tea	Raw vegetables with tofu dip Quick grain salad	Quick parsnip soup Sunburgers Salad with quick carrot dressing Dessert: zucchini bread
Green drink 2 poached eggs on steamed broccoli Essene bread	Quick split pea soup Sunburgers Green salad	Quick fish Sesame rice Salad with mixed vegetables Dessert: carob chip cookies
Buckwheat cereal with nut milk Millet/banana bread Mint tea	Lemon-egg soup with rice Sauerkraut Quick 2-slice buckwheat bread	Quick potato soup Tomato-zucchini sauté Quick avocado/watercress salad with lemon/ soy dressing Dessert: apple sauce
Green drink 2 soft boiled eggs Essene bread with honey-carrot marmalade	Quick gaspacho soup Rice cake with miso/tahini spread and sprouts	Quick miso soup Wild rice and pasta sauté Salad Dessert: sweet treats candies
Super cereal with nut milk Rye/carrot muffin Herbal tonic tea	Wild rice salad Raw vegetables with tofu dip	Lentil tomato soup Pecan/pasta salad Dessert: banana ice cream
Breakfast-in-a-glass	Pecan pasta salad Rice with lentil sauce	Quick borscht Baked chicken with millet Dessert: fresh fruit pudding
Cream of millet cereal with nut milk, soaked currants and sliced banana Calcium tea	Lentil walnut burgers Salad	Curried chicken Salad Dessert: pineapple tofu custard

TIPS FOR PLANNED MENU CHART

The suggested menus on this chart are quick, delicious and nutritionally well-balanced. They incorporate simple menu planning and preparation ideas, and time-saving techniques that are covered in this book, such as:

1. *Protein combining:*
    Combining any of the following categories of foods makes a whole protein, when eaten within 16 hours:
    Seeds and nuts + legumes, such as:
    lentil-walnut burgers
    miso-tahini spread
    sunburgers + split pea soup
    pecan pasta salad + lentil soup or lentil sauce
    Legumes + grains, such as:
    tofu dip + crackers or miso soup + whole grain muffin
    miso/tahini spread + rice cake
    lentil sauce + rice
    Seeds and nuts + grains, such as:
    nut milks on cereal
2. *Making quick blended soups,* such as: quick gazpacho, quick parsnip soup, quick potato soup
3. *Using leftovers creatively*
    Use leftover grain as a creamy cereal the next day, or for a soup or salad such as:
    cream of millet cereal
    wild rice salad
    lemon-egg soup with rice
    Use leftover beans in a soup, salad, or sauce, such as:
    lentil sauce
    Make enough burgers so you have left overs for another meal, such as: lentil-walnut burgers; sunburgers

4. *Pre-prepared dip*

    Make a great dip to use with vegetables, grains, beans, etc. Add water to it to make a sauce. For example:

    miso-tahini spread

    tofu dip

    tahini dip

5. *Avoiding poor combinations*

    Avoid combinations, such as protein + fruit, or protein + starch, with a few exceptions, such as fish + rice; banana + millet or eggs + Essene bread.

6. *To help avoid fresh vegetable waste*

    If you have more vegetables than you need for one meal, plan another meal soon after which incorporates the same vegetables. For example:

    tomato zucchini sauté at one meal

    quick gaspacho soup, using tomatoes and zucchinis at the next.

7. *Use these tips to create your own recipes that are quick, delicious and full of health.*

GLOSSARY

AGAR AGAR (KANTEN)

A gelatinous sea vegetable used like gelatin to make jelled salads and desserts. Agar comes in flake, powder or stick form.

AMARANTH

This grain-like seed is at least 8,000 years old, from the time of the Aztecs. It has been called the "seed sent by God," perhaps because of its super nutritional value: it contains 80% of the USDA of iron, is almost a complete protein and is rich in calcium—three unusual and valuable characteristics for a vegetarian food. It is also rich in fiber, folic acid and phosphorus. Although it is low in gluten, making it virtually non-allergenic, it bakes well, with a nutty, slightly bitter flavor.

ARROWROOT

The finely ground tuberous root of certain plants from the tropical West Indies. Arrowroot has the same uses as cornstarch; i.e. as a thickener for soups, puddings and sauces. Arrowroot is superior to cornstarch because it contains trace minerals and calcium. Cornstarch has no nutritional value, since it is processed.

BRAN

The outer layer, or husk of a grain, such as wheat bran, corn bran, rye bran, oat bran, rice bran, etc. The husk is mostly fiber, the indigestible part of a food. Fiber passes into the lower bowel, or colon, absorbing water and adding bulk to the stool, thereby helping bowel regularity.

BREWER'S YEAST

The micro-organism used by brewers to ferment barley and hops into beer. It is often washed off and sold as a supplement. It is 50% protein, high in B complex vitamins, chromium, selenium, and traces of iron, calcium and potassium.

BUCKWHEAT

A grain-like food, although botanically, it is considered a fruit since its seeds are produced from flowers.

Unlike grains, such as wheat or rice, which contain a bran, germ and endosperm, the buckwheat seed contains only a shell and a kernel inside the shell called a "groat." The groat is the edible portion and is used in the same way grains are used. For example, the groats are ground into flour and used in pancakes or made into buckwheat soba noodles. The groats are roasted (called "kasha") and eaten as a cereal or side dish, used in loaves, stuffings, etc.

When the buckwheat sprouts, it first forms small heart shaped leaves, called buckwheat greens, tender delicacies often used in natural food preparation, especially in a raw foods diet.

Note that buckwheat is not wheat. Therefore, those with wheat allergies can often tolerate buckwheat.

Buckwheat is high in B vitamins, particularly B1, B3, and B6, vitamin A, calcium, phosphorus, iron, potassium, protein (especially the amino acid lysine), complex carbohydrate, and is a good source of rutin, a flavonoid important for capillary integrity.

CANOLA OIL

This oil derived from the rapeseed is primarily monounsaturated, the type of oil that may be beneficial to the heart. Its "light" flavor lends itself for use in baked goods as well as salad dressings, sauces and marinades.

CAROB

A pod found on a tree called the locust honey tree, carob is also called "St. John's Bread" since it is said that St. John fed on carob when in the wilderness. The carob pod can be eaten as is, or ground into a powder and used to give a chocolate-like taste to beverages, brownies, etc.

For real chocolate lovers, carob should not be expected to taste like chocolate. It has its own delicious flavor. It is rich in vitamins A and B complex, as well as many trace minerals, calcium, potassium, phosphorus and magnesium. It costs about the same as chocolate but, unlike chocolate, is naturally sweet, low in calories and low in fat. Be sure to purchase it unsweetened. Sweeten it yourself with pure sweeteners, like honey or barley malt.

COLD-PRESSED OIL

Extracted from a nut, seed or bean with mechanical pressure, rather than high heats. The term "cold pressed" can literally only apply to olive or sesame oil since these are the only two nuts/seeds which yield enough oil without first being heated. Other unrefined oils have been pressed after being heated to a temperature of 200° to 250°. However, cold pressed oils are also produced without the use of chemicals, and are not subjected to a bleaching process. Therefore, be sure your oils say cold pressed on the labels. They can be purchased in health food stores.

DULSE

A red seaweed containing many trace minerals, especially iodine. Dulse can be eaten straight from the bag, or can be added to soups, grain or vegetable dishes, etc. It can be used whole or ground.

ENZYME

A protein occurring naturally throughout the body, acting as a kind of catalyst for all metabolic functions.

HYDROGENATION

A process in which a liquid oil is converted to a hard shortening for longer shelf life and for a different texture. The liquid unsaturated oil is converted to a saturated, or hard form, by chemically forcing it to accept (or saturating it with) hydrogen ions. The process is done with high heats and toxic chemicals, such as methyl silicone and propyl gallate. The mixture is then bleached with chemicals to whiten it to a more commercially saleable product.

KASHA

Roasted buckwheat groats. See "Buckwheat."

KEFIR MILK

A liquid, yogurt-like cultured dairy product. It is made by adding a culture, containing "friendly bacteria"—*Lactobacillus caucasicus*, *Lactobacillus acidophilus* and *Lactobacillus bulgaricus*—to whole, pasteurized milk. These friendly bacteria are said to aid the digestive system, and help restore and maintain well-balanced intestinal flora.

Kefir cheese, made from kefir milk, has the texture and taste of a delicious, rich sour cream.

The label may read "rifek" (kefir spelled backwards) instead of kefir. The generic name "kefir" has been prohibited in New York State, since the product made in New York State does not contain the fermenting, effervescing, alcoholic characteristics of the kefir made in Europe and Asia.

KELP

A seaweed, usually ground to a powder and used as a salt substitute, since it has a salty flavor. It is high in natural iodine and trace minerals. It will add a darker color to the foods to which it is added.

KOMBU

A brown seaweed, used in Japanese and natural food cooking.

KUZU OR KUDZU

A natural root starch used as a superb thickener and jelling agent in natural food cooking. It is also said to contain fine medicinal properties. Entire books have been written on the value of kudzu.

Kudzu is a vine from the Orient, introduced to the U.S. in 1876. There it was praised in the South, where it helped prevent soil erosion, revitalized the soil and made an excellent forage crop. The initial praise quickly died down, however, as the fast-growing vine seemed to take over, engulfing telephone poles, abandoned sites, and smothering trees by blocking out the sunlight. It was joked that the way to plant kudzu was to "plant it and run."

Unfortunately, the value of the kudzu root has not been acknowledged in this country. It is harvested with great expense and difficulty in the Orient and sold in Oriental and natural food stores as small white chunks packaged in clear plastic bags, usually labeled "kuzu."

LIVE FOODS

Unprocessed, uncooked foods in their natural, whole state, such as sprouts. Live foods still contain and impart to you the "breath of life."

MISO

Fermented soybean paste, or soybean plus grain paste (such as rice or barley miso). It is a dark paste that is packaged in a clear, plastic bag or in a tub container. Like yogurt, miso is high in beneficial bacteria and enzymes which aid digestion and food assimilation and help reduce the negative effects of antibiotics.

Miso is used in natural food cooking in soups, sauces, etc. It is extremely salty, as salt is used in the fermenting process along with koji (a starter) and water.

NUT MILK

A milky liquid made by blending nuts and seeds, or nut butters, with water. It can be used in place of milk in any recipe and is high in protein, vitamins and minerals.

NORI

A seaweed, used in Oriental and natural food cooking.

ORGANICALLY GROWN

Organically grown food is food grown without the use of pesticides or artificial fertilizers, and grown in soil whose humus and mineral content is increased by additions of organic matter and natural mineral fertilizers. It is food that has not been treated with preservatives, hormones, antibiotics, etc.

QUINOA (pronounced "KEEN-wah")

Quinoa was one of three staple foods of the Incas of South America. This grain-like food is high in protein, magnesium, potassium, iron, zinc and fiber. It looks like a cross between sesame seeds and millet; it has a subtle, nutty taste, a delicate, light texture, cooks easily and quickly (about 15 minutes) and is virtually non-allergenic.

REJUVELAC

Fermented beverage drained off soaked grain, usually soft pastry wheat, which has been soaked in water overnight or longer. Rejuvelac is high in vitamins E, B, and K and enzymes. It is a predigested food so it may aid digestion and provide friendly bacteria for the colon.

SATURATED FAT

Except for coconut and palm oils, saturated fats are found only in animal protein, and are usually hard at room temperature.

SEA SALT

This salt from sea water, dried naturally in the sun, does not contain additives to make it flow freely, as does refined salt. In addition, sea salt is only 75% sodium chloride, containing other minerals as well as sodium. Therefore, it is more balanced than common table salt, which is pure sodium chloride.

SHOYU or Soy Sauce

The liquid that results from fermenting soybeans, roasted cracked wheat, salt and well water.

SPROUTS

The shoots of plants, such as alfalfa, mung, lentil, etc. They are high in enzymes, vitamins, minerals, protein and life force.

TAHINI

Sesame seed paste, or sesame seed butter, made by grinding sesame seeds. It is similar to peanut butter, but is made with sesame seeds instead of peanuts. Peanut butter is more difficult to digest, and is often contaminated with a mold which has been found to be cancer-causing.

Use tahini as a spread on bread or crackers, or make a sauce, dip or dressing with it. Blend it with water and honey for a drink. Add it to oatmeal or other grains. Put it in candies or desserts.

TAMARI or Soy Sauce

Originally the liquid that resulted from fermenting soybeans, salt and koji (a mold starter). Sometimes it has wheat added, to alter the flavor.

TEMPEH

Fermented cooked soy beans. It is made by adding a *rhizopus* culture to lightly cooked soybeans, and letting them stand in a warm place overnight. The culture partially digests the beans, and binds them together with a fine, white mycelium.

TOFU

Soybean curd, first made in China over 2,000 years ago and used as a primary source of protein in the East Asian diet.

Tofu is the white block that sits in open containers of water in Oriental or vegetable markets. It also comes in a package, refrigerated in health food stores. The packaged tofu is better, because it is less likely to be contaminated from sitting out in the open. However, make sure it contains no toxic additives.

To make tofu, soybeans are soaked overnight, ground into a purée and cooked in steam. The soy milk is squeezed from the pulp, and nigari (seawater extract) is added as a solidifier. The milk separates into curd and whey. The whey is ladled off and the curd is put into a tray lined with cheesecloth and then pressed with weights.

Tofu is used in natural food cooking as a source of protein. It is a great base for dips, ice creams, pies, blender drinks, etc. Entire books have been written on the uses of tofu. The simplest way to begin using it is to cut it in chunks and add it to soups.

TRITICALE

A hybrid grain, resulting from crossing wheat and rye seeds. It has 16.4% more protein than most of the cereal grains. Although it is a cross-breed, it can reproduce itself. Because of its high amino acid balance, it has a biological value close to that of eggs and meat—closer than rye or wheat by themselves.

UMEBOSHI

Plums pickled in brine. The plums are sprinkled with salt, arranged in layers in wooden kegs, earthenware crocks, or concrete vats lined with fiberglass. Then they are compressed by a layer of straw mats, a wooden lid and large stones. For 1–2 months the pickling process is carried out by salt and some fermentation enzymes which cause the production of lactic acid, one of the most important components of umeboshi, together with citric acid.

Umeboshi vinegar is delicious on grains and vegetables, and umeboshi paste may be used in place of salt in sauces and dressings or as a topping for corn on the cob.

UNSATURATED FAT

Unsaturated fatty acids are usually liquid at room temperature, and are primarily derived from vegetables, nuts or seeds, such as sunflower or sesame oil. It is thought that monounsaturated fats such as olive oil, canola oil, almonds, walnuts and avocados are less likely to contribute fatty deposits in blood vessels than saturated fats such as meat, chicken, whole-milk dairy products and butter.

UNSULFURED

The toxic chemical sulfur dioxide has not been used in the processing of a food that is unsulfured. In the case of dried fruit, sulfur dioxide is often used to enhance and preserve color. The cut fruit is exposed to fumes of burning sulfur, which penetrates the fruit and inactivates the enzymes, preserving the color. For example, sulfured dried apricots are bright orange, whereas unsulfured dried apricots are usually brown. Sulfur fumes combine with water in the dried fruit, forming sulfurous acid, which remains in the fruit and is toxic to humans.

WAKAME

A seaweed, or sea vegetable, used in Oriental and natural food cooking.

WHEATGRASS

Grass grown from the wheat berry. High in enzymes, vitamins, minerals and chlorophyll. The grass is chewed, or juiced with a special juicer.

INDEX

acceptable foods (chart), 54–55
additives, common (chart), 282–285
  toxic, 46–47
aduki beans, 31
agar agar, 6, 292
alcohol
  effects of, 49–50
  "transition" beverage, 50
alfalfa recipes
  croquettes, 180
  sprouts, 31
all-American pizza, 211
allergens, common, 32, 33, 37, 49, 51
almonds, 32
  blanching, 143
  cake, 261
  candies, 253
  frosting, 264
  milk, 143
  oil, 36
  torte, flour-free, 260
aluminum cookware, avoid, 65
amaranth, 29, 292
  muffins, 117
apples, applesauce
  apple pie filling, 265
  apple tarts, easy, 267
  applesauce muffins, 116
  applesauce, raw, 266
arame, 41
arrowroot, thickening agent, 6, 193, 293
artichoke, steamed, 218
aspartame, 45
avocado, 42
  dip, 190
  grapefruit salad, 182
  oil, 36
  sunchoke salad, 178
  watercress salad, 176

baking hints, 108; low heat baking, 111
baking powder, 46
baking soda, 46
banana, 42, 51
  bread, millet, 112
  dressing, 188
  ice cream, dairy-free, 269, 270, 271
  shake, 145, 146
  split, 271
barley, 29, 51; cooking, 223
  cream cereal, 126
  malt, 38
  soup, 163
  water, 153
beans, 31, 41, 51; cooking, 242–245
  combinations, suggested, 244
  iron absorption and, 31
  loaf and wild rice, 248
  protein source, 81
  salad, 249
  soup, 163
  tofu and, 242–250
beef, 35, 51
beets; use raw beets sparingly, 148
  borscht, 171
  sunflower dressing, 187
better butter (butter substitute), 36, 194
beverages, 37, 137–157
blender foods
  salad, 177
  soups, 170–173
  super sauce or gravy, 194
  vegetable dressing, 186
blender, cleaning tips, 280
borscht, raw, 171
bran, 293
brazil nuts, 32
breads, 108–117, 277
  buckwheat, 111
  cornmeal, 111

breads *continued*
  Essene, 109
  rye, 110
  storing breads, 277
  sprouted grain, raw, 109
  whole wheat, 110
brewers yeast, 293
brilliant Mary, 149
broccoli, steamed, 218
broth, potato peel, 157
brown barley cream cereal, 126
brown rice, 229
brownies, carob, 256
buckwheat, 29, 293; cooking, 223
  bread, 111
  pancakes, 132
  pasta and sunchokes, 241
  porridge, 124
  sprouts, 31
bulgur (cracked wheat), 29; cooking,
    223
  bulgur salad, 233
burgers, vegetarian
  lentil walnut, 247
  sunflower, 212–213
butter, 36
  "better butter," 36, 194

cabbage, 41
caffeine, 50
cake recipes
  almond, 261
  vanilla, 261
  carrot, 259
  rum, 261
calcium tea, 156
calories, 72–73
candy recipes
  almond, 253
  carob mint, 253
  carob orange, 253
  quick, 253
  sesame marzipan, 253
  sweet treats, 254
canola oil, 36, 294
carob, 6, 58, 294
  bananas, frozen, 269
  brownies, 256
  chip cookies, 257

filling for graham crackers, 255
frosting, Eva's, 263
mint kisses, 253
mint sauce, 272
mocha sauce, 272
orange candies, 253
orange sauce, 272
powder, 38
sauce, 272
shake, 145
carrot recipes
  cake, 259
  dressing, 186, 188
  marmalade, gingered, 197
  salad, 176
  soup, 162
cashews, caustic oil in, 32
casserole recipes
  pilaf, 231
  quick vegetable, 210
cayenne pepper, 39, 94
cereals, whole grain, 119–130
  cooking techniques, 121
  improving digestion of, 122
  ingredients, 119–120
cereal recipes
  brown barley cream, 126
  corn meal cream, 126
  cream of grain, 124
  millet, 126
  sprouted rye, 127
  sprouted wheat, 127
  super, 128–129
  thermos, 127
  30–minute, 125
charts, reference
  common food additives, 282–285
  cooking dried beans, 245
  create-a-meal, vegetables, 207–209
  create-a-soup, 165
  enriching recipes, 62–63
  food equivalent measurements, 96–98
  grain cooking, 224–225
  hidden salt, 288–289
  hidden sugars, 286–287
  meal plan, 74
  quick planned menus, 290
  vital foods/foods to avoid, 54–55
cheese, 36
  cheese-rice-nut loaf, 230

cherry breakfast, 144
chestnuts, 32
chia seeds, 32
    sprouts, 31
chick pea dip (hummus), 246
chicken, 199–201
    coq au vin, 200
    curried, 201
    noodle soup, 167
    salad, 249
children, cooking for, 19–20
cinnamon, 51
citrus, 51
chocolate, 51
    chocolate to carob conversion, 58
cholesterol, eggs and, 33
cider vinegar, 39
cocktails, vegetable juice, 147–148
coconut oil, avoid, 49
coffee, 50, 51
colas, 50, 51
cold-pressed oil, 295
compote, dried fruit, 266
conversions, dietary
    chocolate to carob, 58
    milk to "nut milk," 60
    recipes, 56–57
    salt replacements, 58
    sugar to honey, 57
    sugar to molasses, 58
    white flour to whole wheat flour, 59
    white rice to brown rice, 60
cookie recipes
    carob chip, 257
    oatmeal, 258
cooking hints, techniques
    cereals, 121
    chicken, 199–201
    eggs, 135
    fast food, 89–90
    fish, 202
    grains, 219–228
    low heat, 92, 111
    nut milks, 141–142
    pancakes, 131
    pasta, 237–238
    preserve nutrients, 92
    salads, 174–175
    soups, 158–160
    vegetables, 205–209

cookware, recommended, 65
copper cookware, 65
coq au vin, 200
corn, 51
    bread, 111
    cream cereal, 126
    pancakes, 132
corn oil, 49
cottonseed oil, avoid, 49
cranberries
    juice, 152
    relish, 198
cravings, 23–25
    dehydration and, 24
    food sensitivities and, 23
    salty foods and blood sugar, 23
cream of grain cereal, 124
create-a-meal, vegetables, 207–209
create-a-soup, 164–165
croquettes
    alfalfa (raw), 180
    quinoa/potato, 232
cupcakes, 261
currants, 42
curried chicken, 201
curried tofu mayonnaise, 236
custard, pineapple-tofu, 268
cutting board, cleaning, 281

dairy products, 36, 78
    dairy-free banana ice cream, 270
    dairy-free eggnog, 145
    nut milk alternatives, 141–144
dehydration and food cravings, 24
dessert recipes, 251–272
    almond torte, 260
    applesauce, raw, 266
    banana split, 271
    basic vanilla cake, 261
    candies, quick, 253
    carob brownies, 256
    carob chip cookies, 257
    carob graham crackers, 255
    carob mint quick dessert, 271
    carob sauce, basic, 272
    carrot cake, 259
    dried fruit compote, 266
    easy apple tarts, 267
    fresh fruit ice cream (non-dairy), 270

dessert recipes *continued*
  frostings, icings, 262–264
  frozen fruit "lip sticks," 269
  fruit pies, raw, 265
  fruity banana (frozen), 271
  ice cream toppings, 270
  mocha sauce quick dessert, 271
  oatmeal cookies, 258
  pineapple-tofu custard, 268
  popcorn plus, 268
  sweet treats, 264
dietary conversions: See conversions, dietary
digestion, improving, 49, 83–87, 122,
dip recipes, 190–191
  avocado, 190
  guacamole, 190
  hummus (chick pea), 246
  sesame tahini, 191
  spring green, 191
  tahini, 191
  tofu-vegetable, 190
dressings, salad, 184–189
  banana, 188
  beet/sunflower, 187
  blended vegetable, 186
  carrot, 186
  ginger-carrot, 188
  ginger-tahini, 187
  ginger/soy, 186
  honey, 188
  lemon/soy, 185
  mustard, 249
  oil/vinegar, 185, 186
  papaya, 189
  poppy seed, 189
  sesame tahini, 191
  sunflower/beet, 187
  tahini, 191
  tahini-ginger, 187
  tarragon, 187
  tofu-vegetable, 190
  watercress, 188
dried fruit compote, 266
dulse, 41, 58, 295

eating out, 15–16
eggs, 33, 51, 135–136
  poached, 136
  scrambled, 136
  soft boiled, 135
  storing, 277; hints for using, 279
  substitutions for, 61, 141–144
eggnog, dairy-free, 145
endive-watercress salad, 178
enzymes, 295
  sources of, 76
Equal, 45
Essene bread, 109
Eva's bread, 110
Eva's carob frosting, 263

fats, 73
  saturated, 299
  substitutions for, 61
  unsaturated, 302
fenugreek
  fluff, 146
  sprouts, 31
fermented grain water, 154
fermented seed loaf, 213
fiber, sources of, 76
fig, 42
filberts, 32
fish, 34–35, 51, 202–204; "safe" fish, 34
  broiled in lemon sauce, 203
  for one, 203
  noodle soup, 167
  Orientale, 204
flax seeds, 32; oil, 36
flour, wholegrain
  storing, 276
  substitutions, 59–60
flour-free recipes
  almond torte, 260
  pie crust, 264
  vegetable pie, 211
fluff, fenugreek, 146
foo yung, vegetable, 210
food additives, common (chart), 282–285
food combining, 83–87
food, information about
  acceptable foods (chart), 54–55
  allergies, sensitivities, 23, 51
  calories of, 72–73
  converting recipes, 18, 56–57
  cost of, 8

cravings, 23–25
  emotional connections to, 24
  equivalent measurements (chart)
    96–98
  fast cooking techniques, 89–90
  food colors, artificial, 51
  foods to avoid (chart), 54–55
  foods to prepare ahead, 13
  gifts of, 21
  harmful foods, 43–51
  kitchen hints for natural foods,
    275–281
  live foods, 297
  menu planning, 71–77
  organizing preparation of, 12
  preparation, 88–92
  processed foods, effects of, 43
  raw foods and indigestion, 83–84
  shopping hints, 68–70
  spoilage of, 8
  staples, 68–69
  storage of, 12–13, 68
  timing of meals, 85–86
  transition to healthier, 27–42
  travel foods, 17
  visiting, strategies for, 21–22
  vital foods (chart), 54–55
freezer storage, 13–14
frosting, icings, 262–264
  almond, 264
  Eva's carob, 263
  lemon, 263
frozen desserts, 269
fruit fizz, 152
fruit, 38, 78; to quicken ripening, 278
  desserts, frozen, 269, 271
  pies, raw, 265
  salads, 182–183
  sherbet, 270
  toppings, 271

garbanzo beans, 31
  dip (hummus), 246
garlic, 51
garlic press, cleaning, 280
gazpacho soup, 163, 172
ginger recipes
  ginger ale, 153
  gingerbread, 114

ginger-carrot dressing, 188
ginger-carrot marmalade, 197
ginger-tahini dressing or sauce, 187
ginger-soy dressing, 186
goat's milk, 36
golden roasted granola, 130
gomasio, 39
"good, better, best" guide, 24
graham crackers, carob filling for, 255
grains, whole, 29–30, 78, 219–236
  cooking chart, 224–225
  cooking hints for, 219–223
  "enriched," 47
  salads, 233–235
  soup, 163
  storing, 276
  grain water, fermented, 154
  grain water recipes, 153–154
gram equivalents, 94–95
granola recipes
  golden roasted, 130
  pie crust, 267
grapefruit and avocado salad, 182
grater, cleaning tips, 280
gravy recipes
  mushroom, 248
  quick blended, 194
green dip, spring, 191
greens, leafy, 41; storing, 275–276
guacamole dip, 190

herbal teas, 155–156
herbs and spices, 39
hijiki, 41
homogenized milk, 50
honey, 38
  dressing, 188
  in baking, 57
  to liquify crystallized, 278
  to measure, 278
honigar (honey-vinegar beverage), 157
hot mulled juice, 151
hummus, 246
hydrogenation, 295

ice cream, dairy-free, 270
  toppings, 270
icings, 262–264

indigestion, avoiding, 49, 83–87, 122
ingredient labels, 30, 44
ingredients, hidden, 44
Italian tofu and pasta, 240

jams and jellies, 197–198
jars, storing with lids, 279
Jerusalem artichoke (sunchokes)
    and noodles, 241
    salad, 178
juices, 37
    hot mulled, 151

kamut, 30
kanten, 41, 292
kasha, 29, 296
kefir, 36, 296
kelp, 41, 58, 296
kidney beans, 31
kilogram equivalents, 94–95
kitchen equipment, 64–68
kiwi, 42
kombu, 41, 296
kuzu root powder, 185, 192, 297

labels, ingredient, 30, 44
lamb, 35
leek potato soup, 173
leftovers, using creatively, 291
lemons, 278
    egg soup, 169
    frosting, 263
    soy dressing, 185
    to squeeze juice, 278
lentils, 31
    sprouts, 31
    tomato soup, 169
    walnut burgers, 247
liter equivalents, 94–95
loaf recipes
    rice-nut-cheese, 230
    wild rice and bean, 248
low heat baking, 111

macadamia nut, highest in fat, 32
malt, barley, 38

malt, tofu, 146
mango, 42
maple syrup, 38
marinated vegetables, 180
marmalade, carrot, 197
marzipan, sesame, 253
mayonnaise, curried tofu, 236
meal plan chart, 74
meal timing, indigestion and, 85–86
measurement abbreviations, 94; equiva-
    lents, 94–95
meat, 35, 47–48
menu planning 19, 291–292
milk, 51
    almond, 143
    homogenized, 50
    milk to "nut milk" conversion, 60
    pasteurized, 50
    sesame, 144
millet, 29; cooking, 223, 229
    banana bread, 112
    cereal, 126
    flour, 59
milliliter equivalents, 94–95
minerals, sources of, 77
mint refresher (tea), 155
miso, 6, 297
    soup, 168
    tahini spread or sauce, 194
mixed vegetable juice, 149
mocha recipes
    sauce, 272
    shake, 146
mock tabouli (bulgur salad), 234
molasses, 38, 58
MSG (monosodium glutamate), 46
muffin recipes
    amaranth, 117
    applesauce, 116
    corn, 115
mulled juice, 151
mung beans, 31
mushroom gravy, 248
mustard dressing, 249

navy beans, 31
no-tomato tomato sauce, 196
noodles, sunchoke, 241
nori, 298

NutraSweet, 45
nuts, 32
   nut milk, 37, 298, 141–144
   nut-rice-cheese loaf, 230
   protein source, 81
   rancidity and, 32
   storing, 276
   sunny salty snack, 252

oats, 29, 51; cooking, 223
   sprouts, 31
oatmeal, 123
   cookies, 258
oils, 36–37
   cold-pressed, 295
   indigestible, 49
   processed, 48–49
   recommended, 77, 93–94
   storing, 276
   vitamin E helps preserve, 36
   vinegar dressing, 185, 186
omelettes, 135–136
onions, 51
   soup, 167
orange sauce, carob, 272
organically grown, 298
ounce equivalents, 94–95

palm oil, 49
pancakes, 131–134
   buckwheat, 132
   cooking hints, 131
   cornmeal, 132
   potato, 217
   toppings, 132
papaya, 42
   dressing, 189
parasites in pork, fish, 48
parsnip soup, 162
pasta, 237–241
   cooking hints for, 237
   Italian tofu and, 240
   pasta plus, 239
   pecan salad, 241
   serving suggestions, 238
   sunchokes and, 241
   wild rice and, 232
pasteurized milk, 50

peanuts, 32, 51
   oil, 49
peas, 41, 51
   salad, 179
   split, 31
pecans, 32, 51
   pasta salad, 241
persimmon, 42
phenylketonuria (PKU), 45
pie crust recipes
   flour-free, 264
   granola, 267
   quinoa, 233
pie filling recipes
   apple, 265
   mixed dried fruit, 265
pie, vegetable
   flour-free vegetable, 211
   scallion sweet potato, 214
pilaf casserole, 231
pilaf cooking method, 227
pineamile punch, 151
pineapple recipes
   drink variations, 150
   fenugreek shake, 146
   green drink, 150
   protein punch, 149
   tofu custard, 268
pinto beans, 31
pizza, all-American, 211
poached eggs, 136
popcorn, 268
poppy seed dressing, 189
pork, 48, 51
porridge, buckwheat, 124
potatoes, 51; See also sweet potatoes
   herbed potatoes, 217
   leek soup, 173
   pancakes, 217
   potato flour substitutions, 60
   potato peel broth, 157
   quinoa croquettes, 232
   soup, 162, 173
poultry, 35
processed foods, 47
   alternatives to toxic additives, 47
protein, 77–79
   combining 81, 291, 292
   complete, 81, 122
prune, 42

psyllium seeds, powdered, 185
pudding, sweet potato, 217
pumpkin recipes
  seeds, 32
  spice bread, 113
  sprouts, 31

quick recipes
  blended super sauce or gravy, 194
  candies, 253
  creamy grain or bean soup, 163
  creamy root vegetable soup, 162
  fish for one, 203
  vegetable casserole, 210
quinoa, 29, 298
  pie crust, 233
  potato croquettes, 232

radish, 41
  sprouts, 31
raisin, 42
raw foods, 83–84
  applesauce, 266
  borscht, 171
  fermented seed loaf, 213
  fruit pies, 265
  milk, 37
  spinach soup, 170
  vegetable snacks, 179
  vegetable soup, 161
recipe conversion, 56–57
refrigerator storage, 13–14
rejuvelac (fermented grain water), 154,
  299
relish, cranberry, 198
restaurant dining, 15–16
rice, brown, 29, 229; cooking, 223
  lemon-egg soup, 169
  nut-cheese loaf, 230
  sesame, 230
rice, wild, recipes
  bean loaf, 248
  pasta and, 232
  salad, 236
  stuffing, 215
rice bran syrup, 38
rice flour substitutions, 60
roll recipes

rye, 110
  whole wheat, 110
rum cake, 261
Ruth Duffy's tarragon dressing, 187
rye, 29, 51; cooking, 223
  bread, 110
  sprouts, 31

saccharin, 45
safflower oil, 49
sage brush (chia) seeds, 32
salad dressings, 184–189
salad recipes, 174–183
  alfalfa croquettes, 180
  avocado and grapefruit, 182
  avocado-sunchoke, 178
  avocado-watercress, 176
  bean, 249
  blended, 177
  bulgur, 233
  carrot, 176
  chicken, 249
  endive-watercress, 178
  fruit, 182–183
  grain, 233–235
  grapefruit and avocado, 182
  Jerusalem artichoke, 178
  mock tabouli, 234
  pasta-pecan, 241
  pea, 179
  pecan-pasta, 241
  sunchoke-avocado, 178
  tomato-basil, 177
  tropical delight, 182
  watercress-avocado, 176
  watercress-endive, 178
  wild rice with curried tofu mayon-
    naise, 236
salt, 45–46
  hidden salt in foods (chart), 288–289
  salt replacements, conversion, 58
  sea salt, 39, 29
salt-free sauerkraut, 181–182
saturated fat, 299
sauce recipes, 192–196
  basic carob, 272
  carob mint, 272
  carob orange, 272
  ginger-tahini, 187

miso-tahini, 194
mocha, 272
no-tomato tomato, 196
real tomato, 195
sesame tahini, 191
tahini, 191
tahini-ginger, 187
tahini-miso, 194
tofu-vegetable, 190
tomato, 195–196
vegetable-tofu, 190
sauerkraut, salt-free, 181–182
scallion sweet potato pie, 214
scrambled eggs, 136
scrambled tofu, 250
sea salt, 39, 299
sea vegetables (seaweeds) 37, 41, 58
seasonings, 39
seeds, 32
    loaf, raw fermented, 213
    protein source, 81
    storing, 276
    sunny salty snack, 252
sesame seeds, 32
    marzipan, 253
    milk, 144
    oil, 36
    rice, 230
    tahini dip, sauce or dressing, 191
shake recipes
    banan-almond fig, 146
    carob, 145
    mocha, 146
    pineapple fenugreek, 146
sherbet, fresh fruit, 270
shortening, substitutions for, 61
shoyu, 299
shrimp, 51
side dishes, 216
slippery elm powder, 185
smoothies and shakes, 145–146
snacks and desserts, 251–272
    importance of, 16
    raw vegetable, 178
soft drink recipes, 152–153
soup recipes, 158–173,
    barley, 163
    bean, 163
    blended, 170–173
    borscht, 171

carrot, 162
chicken noodle, 167
fish noodle, 167
gazpacho, 163, 172
grain, 163
leek potato, 173
lemon-egg, 169
lentil-tomato, 169
miso, 168
onion, 167
parsnip, 162
potato, 162, 173
potato leek, 173
quick gazpacho, 163
raw spinach, 170
raw vegetable, 161
rice-lemon-egg, 169
spinach, raw, 170
squash, 162, 171
sweet potato, 171
tomato-lentil, 169
turnip, 162
vegetable, 166
soy beans, 31
soy flour substitutions, 60
soy oil, 36
soy sauce, 39, 58, 93, 299
spelt, 30
spinach soup, raw, 170
spoilage, 8
spread recipes, 192–196
    miso-tahini, 194
spring green dip, 191
sprouted grain recipes
    cereal, 127
    bread, raw, 109
    rye cereal, 127
    wheat cereal, 127
sprouts, 31, 80, 99–107, 299
    how to grow, 100–107
    nutrition of, 99
squash recipes
    soup, 162, 171
    baked, 215
strawberry jam, 197
stuffing, wild rice, 215
sugar, 51
    avoid excess, 45
    hidden sugar in foods (chart),
        286–287

sugar *continued*
  natural sugars, 38
  sugar to honey conversion, 57
  sugar to molasses conversion, 58
sulfur dioxide, avoid, 38, 302
sunburgers, 212–213
sunchoke (Jerusalem artichoke) recipes
  avocado salad, 178
  noodles, 241
sunflower seeds, 32
  almond milk, 143
  beet dressing, 187
  breakfast, 144
  oil, 36
  sunburgers, 212–213
  sprouts, 31
  sunny salty snack, 252
super cereal, 128–129
Sweet 'n Low, 45
Sweet One, 45
sweet potato 41
  pudding, 217
  scallion pie, 214
  soup, 171
sweet treats, 254
sweeteners, 38
  artificial, 45

tabouli (bulgur salad), mock, 234–235
tahini, sesame, 6, 300
  dip, sauce, or dressing, 191
  ginger dressing or sauce, 187
  miso spread or sauce, 194
tamari, 7, 58, 300
tannin, 50
tarragon dressing, 187
tarts, easy apple, 267
tea
  black, 50
  brewing instructions, 155
  herbal, 155–156
  mint refresher, 155
  special calcium, 156
  tummy soother, 156
teff, 30
tempeh, 300
thermos cooking
  cereal, 127
  grain, 226

thickening agents, 185
30–minute cereal, 125
tofu, 7, 250, 300
  beans and, 242–250
  broiled, 250
  Italian, and pasta, 240
  malt, 146
  mayonnaise, curried, 236
  pineapple custard, 268
  scrambled, 250
  storing, 276
  vegetable dip, sauce, or dressing, 190
tomatoes, 51
  basil salad, 177
  lentil soup, 169
  Provencal, 216
  sauce, 195–196
topping recipes
  for fruit, 271
  for ice cream, 270
  for popcorn, 268
torte, almond, flour-free, 260
transition to healthier foods, 27–42,
    53–55
treats, sweet, 254
triticale, 301; cooking, 223
tropical delight salad, 182
tummy soother tea, 156
turnip soup, 162

umeboshi, 301
unsaturated fat, 302
unsulfured, 302
utensils, 64–68
  hints for cleaning, 280

vanilla cake, 261
vegetables, 37, 77, 205–218
  casserole, quick, 210
  cooking tips, 205
  dressing, blended, 186
  foo yung, 210
  how to clean, 275
  juice cocktails, 147–149
  marinated, 180
  pie, flour-free, 211
  root soup, creamy, 162
  sauteed, 206

snacks, raw, 178
soup, 166
soup, raw, 161
steamed, 206
vegetarian menu planning, 79, 80–82
vinegar, apple cider, 39
beverage, 157
visiting, strategies for, 21–22
vital foods (chart), 54–55
vitamins, sources of, 77
vitamin E helps preserve oils, 36

wakame, 41, 302
walnuts, 32, 51
lentil burgers, 247
oil, 36
water, grain (beverage), 153
waterchestnuts, 41
watercress recipes
avocado salad, 176
dressing, 188
endive salad, 178

wheat, whole, 29, 51; cooking, 223
bread, 110
flour, uses of, 59
sprouts, 31
wheatgrass, 139, 302
white flour to whole wheat flour conversion, 59
white rice to brown rice conversion, 60
wild rice recipes
bean loaf, 248
pasta and, 232
salad with curried tofu mayonnaise, 236
stuffing, 215
withdrawal symptoms, 23

yam, 41
yeast, 51
yogurt, 36

zucchini bread, 113